Sweetie Drives
On
Chemo Days

John P. Schulz

For Maria —

Every Thing is going to be all right

John P. Schulz

Sweetie Drives On Chemo Days

Facing Cancer Treatments with Humor and Optimism

John P. Schulz

Sweetie Drives on Chemo Days
Facing Cancer Treatments with Humor and Optimism

ISBN 978-0-9909746-1-1

interior & cover design, recipes by Dekie Hicks
cover photography courtesy:
Chris Ozment chrisozmentphotography.com
Bill Land

Wheredepony Press
Rome, GA
www.wheredeponypress.com

printed in the U.S.A.

After all of the changes in my voice mechanisms due to throat cancer, even though I can talk, I can't laugh out loud. Now a laugh comes out like the wind through the pines.
This time of year I laugh a lot, so when you hear the wind blowing through the tree tops, you are hearing my voice.
Smile, please, join in the hilarity. Throw your arms in the air, laugh out loud and say, "Hey, John." And do it a lot. I have spoken.

➤**John P. Schulz**
Sweetie Drives on Chemo Days

For Dekie
My loving caregiver, trucking buddy,
wife, and best friend

Acknowledgements

Thanks to Doctors Robert King and Matt Mumber of the Harbin Clinic in Rome, Georgia, and to Doctors Kristin Higgins and Nabil Saba of the Winship Cancer Institute of Emory University in Atlanta, Georgia. A special thanks to Doctor Amy Chen of the Emory Clinic, who worked magic on me and then became my cancer shepherd.

Thanks also to Meryl Kaufman and Beth Seelinger, brilliant and empathetic speech therapists and to Physicians Assistants/Nurse Practioners Ulrike Gorgens and Sharon Etris, and all of the countless nurses, technicians, and behind-the-scenes medical personnel who make the whole system run right!

I also wish to thank Marsha Atkins, David Hightower, Joel Todino, Jane B. Schulz, and Robert Hicks for their supportive editorial guidance. Mary de Wit, Sylvia Eidson, and Diana Smithson offered valuable insight into their personal cancer journeys and allowed their words to be included here.

Table of Contents

Index of Recipes

Foreword

At the end of my first visit to the cancer clinic, they gave me a book. I was happy to get the book because I thought it would answer my questions and calm my fears. I brought the book home, made a cup of coffee, and sat down to read and to calm my concerned and fearful mind.

The book was a disappointment. I read some of it, scanned the rest of it, and then threw it aside and went outside to work in my flower bed and meditate. My questions went unanswered and I was left to deal with my fears and other concerns on another level. To help ease my mind I started a journal. I decided that if I had to find my own answers I would keep track of the process.

I found that writing out my thoughts and feelings every day or so helped me to deal with both past and present concerns. I entered the maze of cancer treatments with an open mind and with a high level of curiosity. After a while, after paying attention to what was happening in my life on physical, clinical, and psychological levels, and after having countless discussions with fellow cancer victims, I decided to approach the cancer experience with the goal of writing the book *that I would have liked to have received when I first found out that I had cancer.* I wanted a book for care givers and friends of cancer victims that would also help them to understand.

That is why I wrote this book. I wanted to help others who are just finding out that they have cancer by presenting some of the information that I learned during my own experiences. I also was able to grasp several concepts that were valuable to me at the time and which have enriched my life since. Looking back, the concepts seemed simple but before my cancer experience, they were unreachable. Of course, I did not go through this experience alone; my wife, Dekie, was there with me as my primary caregiver. She gained insights into the caregiver's role, and was kind enough to write about these in the final chapter of this book.

The cancer experience left me with several battle scars which I will tell about, but it also left me with an enriched outlook on life. I am a firm believer in the magic involved in approaching adversities such as this with optimism, humor, and an overall good attitude. We can learn optimism and we can choose our own attitude.

> ➤ John P. Schulz

The wind was against them now, and Piglet's ears streamed behind him like banners as he fought his way along, and it seemed hours before he got them into the shelter of the Hundred Acre Wood and they stood up straight again, to listen, a little nervously, to the roaring of the gale among the treetops.

"Supposing a tree fell down, Pooh, when we were underneath it?"

"Supposing it didn't," said Pooh after careful thought.

"What day is it?"
"It's today," squeaked Piglet.
"My favorite day," said Pooh.

➤**A.A. Milne**

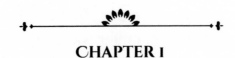

CHAPTER 1

Hello

Hello,

My name is John and I'm a cancer survivor.

Well, so far, anyway.

You just never know what is coming at you.

I think it's interesting that during the same time I had throat cancer, Christopher Hitchens had throat cancer and Michael Douglas had throat cancer. What happened to the three of us? Hitchens died, I had my voice box removed, and Douglas played Liberace in a movie. Do you see what I mean? You just never know what is coming at you.

The good thing is that a cancer diagnosis is not the absolute harbinger of death that it once was. I am one of the first Baby Boomers, having been born in 1945. All my life—until only a very few years ago—I associated the word "cancer" with the word "death." That's the way it was in my formative years. But things are changing. There is a lot of hope around these days and that is what I am writing about—hope, optimism, humor, and survival.

I can remember seeing a John Wayne movie, "The Shootist" (1976), in which the doctor looked at the Wayne character and said, "You have a cancer." Everyone who watched that movie at the time knew from the sound of those words that the character was as good as dead and didn't have long to perform good works.

But attitudes, treatments, and perceptions have changed since the cowboy days. Cancer diagnosis and treatment techniques are changing the idea that the words "cancer" and "death" are always synonymous. After an ultrasound exam at Emory Hospital several months after my laryngectomy and tumor removal, a very nice lady doctor said, "Oh, I'm so sorry, it's cancer. I prayed that it would not be, but it is." I thought about it and grinned at her, answering, "Well, pray again and thank the Lord you found it. Now we can do something about the situation."

That's my attitude. My attitude is that I'm not going to worry or be sad about things. I'm going to get on with it and do something about whatever is wrong with me. I'm not going to worry about tomorrow or the next day, I'm going to take what is going on right now and deal with it. Tomorrow is another day. It always has been and it always will be.

Just to let you know before you go much farther, I am not a doctor or a scientist or a preacher. I'm one of those strange people who ended up with an English degree. I am a writer—one who spends his time studying surroundings and people and happenings—ending up with stories and reports of those observations. Basically, all I know about cancer is that it is caused by body cells doing things that they are not supposed to do. It is about crazy wild cells that kill or otherwise take over good cells which behave properly. It is important to catch and treat the disease in

2

its early stages.

When I was first diagnosed with throat cancer in 2010, I had no idea of what was going on or what was going to happen to me. I don't think I was afraid of dying but I do remember being totally clueless as to what the treatment would consist of. I had heard stories of the terrible things that cancer treatments did to you, like making your hair fall out and making you feel terrible, but I had no idea as to what the treatments consisted of. I had known, or known of, people who had been through cancer treatments, but there was really no one with whom I could talk about it. Actually, I guess I could have found someone to talk to but I wouldn't have known what questions to ask.

Looking back, I noticed my doctors I always asked me if I had any questions. I realized later that they would perfunctorily answer any questions (I assume they are required to) but there was never any volunteered information. Because of this, every process that I was exposed to was a brand new learning experience.

For the technicians who performed the processes, I think it was all rather automatic, similar to a mechanic changing car oil all day long. Not to say that the technicians weren't well-educated, efficient, and very, very nice. The automation was just a feeling that I found interesting and grinned about. I approached all processes with an open mind, without fear, and with a bantering attitude shared with the people who worked on me. My thoughts were (and still are) "If I have to be here anyway, it may as well be pleasant."

One thing that I observed and really appreciated about

the cancer experience was the empathy I received from those around me. Most of my friends and family had little or no idea of what was going to happen to me either and they were understandably concerned. At the beginning of the treatments I didn't feel bad and I didn't really think I deserved all of the consideration and care that I was getting from those who loved me or held me in other high regard. I did come to enjoy and be grateful for the attentions of so many kind people as the treatments progressed and I felt worse.

The main concept that I gained through my experiences with cancer treatment is the importance of maintaining a good attitude. The treatments are grueling at best; trying at all costs to be cheerful and accepting becomes most important. A lot of time is spent in waiting rooms with people from all walks of life who are undergoing similar tribulations. I was able to observe and interact with quite a number of these people.

During my first radiation ritual, I had several talks with David, a redneck drywall hanger who had stage-four lung cancer and was going through radiation and severe chemotherapy. He was a happy-go-lucky joke and story teller who just took things as they came. I enjoyed talking with David, but I felt sorry for him because he just looked terrible, he obviously felt terrible, and I guessed that he wouldn't live long. I was wrong. Two years later I saw David at Home Depot and I hardly recognized him. He was a happy picture of health.

Don't get me wrong, though, I'm not saying that you are definitely not going to die and that you will make it through the treatments and be happy ever after. I've known a lot of people who died from cancer. I have also known many more people who made it through the treatments and lived on, resuming their lives. I also know that your odds of surviving are better now than they have ever been.

You just never know.

I'm going to tell you what happened to me and what I learned about the cancer treatment process. Please be aware that I am not a doctor. I am not a scientist or even science-oriented but I do have a lot of information to pass on.

"Man often becomes what he believes himself to be. If I keep on saying to myself that I cannot do a certain thing, it is possible that I may end by really becoming incapable of doing it. On the contrary, if I have the belief that I can do it, I shall surely acquire the capacity to do it even if I may not have it at the beginning."

➤**Mahatma Gandhi**

"Laughter and tears are both responses to frustration and exhaustion. I myself prefer to laugh, since there is less cleaning to do afterward."

➤**Kurt Vonnegut**

CHAPTER 2

Finding Out

"It's malignant." Those words bring all sorts of reactions. If it's the first time you ever heard these words applied to you, well, you just don't know how to react.

"Oh God, I have cancer."

"Am I going to die?"

"How am I going to tell my wife (husband, children, mother, father, or friends).

"How am I going to pay for it?"

"Will I be able to keep my job?"

The list goes on until all of the panic questions are asked—and you realize that there are no immediate answers. At this point the best way to handle things is to use my favorite mantra. Say it over and over until it becomes real:

"Everything is going to be all right."

Say it again:

"Everything is going to be all right."

The statement has a calming effect. It is optimistic. This is the first step to taking an optimistic approach to dealing with cancer. Say it over and over. Convince yourself that:

"Everything is going to be all right."

After thinking about things for a day or two, my attitude started to change. My thoughts went from, "Oh God, I have cancer" to, "OK, I have cancer. Let's see what happens next. Maybe it's not the worst thing in the world. I can make it through this. I can make it through anything if I set my mind to it."

My thinking had started to move from the negative to the positive. I decided that I was **not** going to let this situation get me down. I decided that I would take whatever was coming at me with optimism. "I'm Superman," I told myself, "I can take anything they give me." I had no idea what I was headed for. All I really knew was that whatever it was would make me feel bad and would make my hair fall out. I can see how little I knew and how a concept or two would have made things easier for me and for those around me.

I now know that there is a treatment that may be self-administered. The one which deals with optimism and attitude. A positive attitude helps with curing. Optimism relieves stress and therefore is also an aid in the healing process.

A positive attitude may be looked at as the belief that everything is for the best and the knowledge that the treatments, no matter how difficult, will come to an end sooner or later with positive results. This attitude deals with knowing that after the treatments are over, you will soon feel better and regain your well-being. There's always a chance that you won't make it but even that reality will be easier to deal with if you maintain a good attitude.

The following steps can help with a positive attitude:

8

Keep a Calendar

1. Keep a calendar that shows the dates of scheduled treatments.

2. Mark off every treatment and make a note of how many are left.

3. Be positive. Each morning when you look at the calendar instead of saying, "Oh, Crap, I've got 20 more treatments to go, I'll never make it" say, "Oooooh! I only have 20 more treatments. Tomorrow it will be 19. I can do it."

4. Always focus on the good side. If there is no good side, invent one.

Keep a Journal

1. Write in it every day. Randy Warley, a psychologist friend of mine, told me that it is better to write the journal by hand rather than type it. He maintains that the act of writing by hand makes the project more special. If need be, you can always transcribe the information to a computer. I actually found myself keeping my journal notes on the notebook app on my iPhone. Picking out the words one letter at a time on the phone slowed me down and helped me to think things through.

2. In your journal, remember to focus on the daily countdown.

3. You should not only keep a record of what happened but also of how you felt about those occurrences.

Remember that optimism is the main part of the positive attitude. Optimism is the concept that gives us our mantra:

"Everything is going to be all right."

9

One of my favorite rhymes that always makes me giggle when things are going wrong or I find myself becoming uptight is this:

> When in trouble, when in doubt
> Run in circles, scream and shout.

Reciting this poem always makes me smile because it somehow helps me to realize the futility of panicking or feeling down about things. Sometimes (when there's no chance of anyone hearing me) I like to yell out the poem and then quietly follow it with,

"Everything is going to be all right."

Optimism is a concept and a practice which can be learned. You will get better with practice. I am naturally optimistic but if that's not the case in your situation, don't despair; you can learn to be optimistic.

Optimism basically involves looking for the good in every situation, no matter how bad it gets. If you are finding a situation hard to handle, stop and ask yourself, "Where is the good in this situation?" Sometimes finding the good is a difficult task but there is usually something, even if it is spiritual. One of the best things you can do is to transfer the optimism to those around you. Optimism is contagious. For instance, one of my sons is so sensitive and caring that he would be sad and somber, worrying about his dad's cancer. I had to keep reassuring him that things would turn out well in the end and that the treatments weren't going to ask more of me than I could give.

I had a hard time transferring the optimism but after a month or two he got the message and his attitude lightened up. Now we can look back and laugh about it.

When you find out that you have cancer, remember that there are many support groups to help with your needs. All you have to do is ask. Also remember that your friends and loved ones will prove to be more supportive if you exhibit a positive attitude and optimism. I think that as soon as you find out what is going on with your treatments, you will worry less about it than will those around you. Things are funny that way.

When you find out that you have cancer, get on the positive side and accept that you will soon be on a difficult regimen but that it is a finite regimen and will be over with sooner or later. Accept that you are entering a phase of your life that will allow you to live—to survive. Practice positivism.

In the writing of this book I am including some of the journal notes that I wrote on my iPhone as time went by. These will be at the end of each chapter (or within the chapter if relevant). Here are the notes from when I found out that the operation had not gotten all of the cancerous growth and that I had malignant tumors—after the ultrasound: (This was six months after the operation to remove the throat cancer and the tumors on my carotid artery—I was a veteran already when this happened).

FROM THE JOURNAL:

The idea that cancer is a death sentence is way prevalent. The doctor has no other option, I think, than to act sensitive and prayerful. It's probably her best defense for those who would overreact.

I am of the opinion that if we have really good people helping, cancer can be beaten and also that there was no way for the surgeon to get all of the big tumor. What they were looking at today was right in the carotid area where the tumor was. It only makes sense that some of it was left in there.

But the tumors are extremely small. They couldn't even see them, it was just that the CT scan told them something had changed. I also think it is way cool that they have a tumor board. I like that. I told her my vote would be to cut it out.

She said that I did have a most important vote in the decision. She loved my attitude.

Absolutely. "From the moment you're born, you are in danger"— T. Jefferson.

I should have told the woman that they couldn't do much more worse than take out my voice box and leave a hole in my throat. How am I supposed to feel about such as that? If I can handle the hole in my *throat, the other stuff should be easy.*

I hope it is something they can cut, otherwise it will be chemo would be my guess. It's not widespread right now and I'll bet those people are the best ever.

Friends and caregivers need to know this:

Here is one of the most important concepts I have to give. ***People who are undergoing treatment for cancer are almost always showing the effects of the treatment rather than the effects of the cancer.*** I wish that I had realized this years ago. I wish, at least, that I had known it when I started my treatments. Oh, well. At least I know it now and I can share the information at every opportunity.

Friends and caregivers must come to know that during the treatment period you may be feeling rather poorly on a physical level but that you don't have to feel poorly on the mental side of things. If you get tired, laugh about it and go take a nap. Enjoy the fact that this is a phase in your life in which it is perfectly acceptable to take a nap any time you wish. This is not saying that you need to stay in bed, just that it's all right to take a nap. At other times, you need to be as active as possible. One of the easy pitfalls to enter is that of boredom. If you don't feel like doing something, forego it, but if you feel like it, don't let the fact that you are taking treatments get in the way of any activities that are pleasurable to you.

From Sylvia:

Am not sure how I feel about your statement that people going through treatment mostly show the signs of the treatments rather than the disease.

Many who are not treated until late stage, or not treated at all—those who are terminal—look awful. Could show you a pic of my ex who died of untreated lung cancer—a terrible sight.

Boredom comes from day after day of feeling too bad to do anything. Can't read, can't pay attention long enough to watch television. There is nothing you can do and that is boring

Roasted Brussel Sprouts with Pecan Vinaigrette

½ lb. brussel sprouts
2 T. butter, melted
½ t. salt
2 T. olive oil
½ c. chopped pecans
1 t. yellow mustard
1 t. vinegar
2 t. honey

Toss sprouts with melted butter and salt. Roast at 400 20-25 minutes. Meanwhile, heat olive oil in skillet over medium heat. Toast pecans until fragrant. Whisk mustard, vinegar, honey together and pour over pecans. Toss sprouts with dressing.

"It's snowing still," said Eeyore gloomily.
"So it is."
"And freezing."
"Is it?"
"Yes," said Eeyore. "However," he said, brightening up a little, "we haven't had an earthquake lately."

➤**A.A. Milne**

"Tell them what you told me the other day about your new problem: If they can fix it, they will; if they can't, we'll deal with it."

➤**Jane B. Schulz**

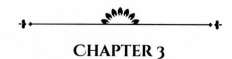

CHAPTER 3

The Oncologists

Depending on how you find out the nature of your problem—from your family doctor, some other specialist, or as in my case, an ENT—you will be referred to an oncologist.

An oncologist is a doctor who specializes in cancer treatment. There are different types of oncologists, depending on specialty, such as radiation onology or chemotherapy oncology. Going to visit the oncologist is the first step in the cancer treatment journey. This is where you get poked and prodded and examined and explored. The doctor will more than likely schedule a scan. This will probably conclude your first visit to the oncologist.

At this point, remember:

"Everything is going to be all right."

It is important also to know that every person who has cancer has his or her own type of cancer and his or her own special set of circumstances. This is why the oncologists are so important. Each case is approached in an individual manner. The treatments may seem the same from person to person, but they are quite individualized. The oncologists are very careful and most meticulous.

My surgeon sent me to two oncologists, one for chemotherapy and another for radiation. The chemo people had my ears checked by a hearing specialist to make sure that my hearing would not be affected by the chemicals. When the auditory specialist found a hearing deficiency, my chemo doctor switched the chemicals in order to avoid taking any chances that they would further harm my hearing.

Initial visits to the oncologists are not unpleasant. These are exploratory visits that concentrate on finding all possible problematic situations and designing a program of treatment to deal with them. After the treatments begin, these doctors will monitor them as they progress by checking the patient's overall well-being and response levels. I believe common practice is for the patient to visit the doctor about once a week during the treatment period. This is definitely true in most cases I have seen for radiation treatments. The visits are mainly to check the progress of the treatments as well as the patient's well-being.

There are so many different kinds of cancers and cancer treatments that we can only make generalized guesses as to what will happen in any individual case. In dealing with so many variables, exceptions to the rules seem to become the rule. The job of the oncologist, then, becomes that of finding, analyzing, and categorizing the variables in order to devise, implement, and monitor a treatment plan.

Since I had throat cancer and the radiation was expected to be invasive, the radiation people called for a feeding tube to be inserted into my stomach. I think this was the most painful procedure of the entire cancer treatment process. Even though the procedure was painful, I realized that my body was healing quickly as I noticed an absence of pain while I was bringing in fire wood about a week or so after the installation. The pain had subsided without my paying attention. Pain is like that. The funny thing was that I refused to use the feeding tube and cursed it soundly every day that it was in my body. I was damned if I would quit swallowing. Determination is important during these treatments.

I think that the status of my radiation oncologist allowed her to get anything she wanted whenever she pleased. Whatever scans, tests, or procedures are needed to make sure the diagnosis and treatment plan(s) are thorough will be quickly and efficiently scheduled.

Here is a journal entry written the day before my treatments began. I think I was more concerned with the pain and inconvenience of the tube than with the scope of the treatments. I was also concerned with how what I later called "the regimen" would work out. I had no idea what was going to happen with my body or my time. I think I was as worried about Sweetie as she was of me.

FROM THE JOURNAL:

Feb 2013

Well, I feel fine this evening. My stomach has even stopped hurting. I didn't even realize it had stopped hurting until I found myself carrying in some fire wood. Isn't it funny how that sort of thing happens?

❖

They are using Carboplatin also called paraplatin or Carbo and Paclitaxel, also called Taxol.

These are given intravenously once a week along with other things to prevent nausea, allergic reactions, etc.

One of the things they tell me is that I should avoid causing a pregnancy for at least 6 months after chemotherapy ends. At my age I think I will be able to deal with this.

The radiation episodes are scheduled for 7:30 a.m. Dekie is going to ride with me tomorrow morning to make sure I can handle it. At that point I plan to do the driving myself or ask a friend or hire a driver. I don't want to wear her out. Sweetie can drive on chemo days. After radiation I can be back around 10 to work my guys and keep up with my customer obligations as well as my financial obligations. I hope all of this will work. I have a good job list going on and you all know how wonderful my clients are. (referring to my landscape maintenance customers)

I used the mantra,
"Everything is going to be all right."
And in the end, after several months or a year or so, everything was all right.

The doctors work hard at trying to keep their patients morale up. I wrote a little poem in my journal about one of the conversations with my radiation doctor.

SECURITY

The old man stood at the podium.

From the audience a request was made, "Tell us of security."

The old man looked down at his folded hands

and thought for a moment.

His face brightened and he raised a forefinger as he began to
            speak

"I had a lump on my shoulder about here,"

he said, pointing to a place just to the base of his neck.

"I was told by an excellent doctor

that I needed to receive radiation applications

to treat a tumor on my carotid artery." He paused.

"That's the artery that takes the blood to the brain,"

he explained.

"I felt secure.

I felt secure in knowing that I was being treated

by very competent people.

I was not afraid."

The old man looked up and smiled.

"But the doctor said..." he continued,

"The doctor said, 'By the way,

There's a chance that your artery will explode.'

And I replied, "Ooooh, that sounds painful."

The doctor laughed and said, 'If it were to explode

It would be sudden and you would not feel a thing'."

The old man looked at the people and smiled,

"So I entered treatment

21

with the secure feeling that if my carotid artery exploded
I wouldn't feel a thing.
And that's about as much security as I ever expect to have."

From Sylvia

In my case before radiation I had to visit a dentist and have a plastic mouth guard to cover my teeth, one for upper and one for lower. I had to wear them during radiation. Point being—depending on the type of cancer, location, etc. each patient's treatment is different.

When your oncology nurse suggests that you take an anti-depressant, follow her advice. You may not feel depressed and resist the meds, but really the doctors know best in this case. It is easy to withdraw from the anti-depressant after your chemo/radiation ends. The professionals will tell you how.

Turkey Cheeseburger Meatloaf

7 slices bacon
1 lb. ground turkey
1 c. shredded sharp cheddar cheese
1 egg
½ small onion, diced
¼ c. breadcrumbs
2 T. Worchestershire sauce
dash cayenne pepper, paprika
salt to taste

glaze ingredients:
¼ c. ketchup
2 T. yellow mustard
2 T. brown sugar
dash Worchestershire sauce

Cook bacon until crisp, drain, and crumble. Pour off most of the grease, saute onions in remaing bacon fat. Add onions and remaining ingredients to turkey. Mix well and form into a ball or loaf. Mix glaze ingredients and spoon evenly over meat. Bake at 350° 45 minutes to one hour. Allow to rest 10-15 minutes before slicing.

Faux Taters (mashed cauliflower)

1 head cauliflower, broken into florets
½ c. whipped cream cheese
1 t. seasoned salt, such as Lowery's
buttermilk

Cook cauliflower in boiling water until tender; drain very thoroughly. Mash with the cream cheese and seasoned salt, or run through food processor. Put mixture in saucepan and heat through, adding buttermilk until desired consistency.

"Write it on your heart that every day is the best day in the year."

> **Ralph Waldo Emerson**

"I, not events, have the power to make me happy or unhappy today. I can choose which it shall be. Yesterday is dead, tomorrow hasn't arrived yet. I have just one day, today, and I'm going to be happy in it."

> **Groucho Marx**

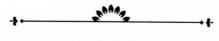

CHAPTER 4

The Scan

I have now had four different kinds of scans, CT scan (computed tomography—CAT scan is no longer correct), PET scan (positron emission tomography), MRI (magnetic resonance imaging) and ultrasound. I'm sure there are more types of scans. There is nothing there to be afraid of. If you want to know a lot of details about the scans, get out your fancy phone and check Wikipedia. There's no sense in my even trying to give you the information when you have that research option. And to do so would slow down the reading cadence!

The CT scan is a relatively simple thing. Doctors and hospitals use this scanning process to check out all sorts of maladies. The scan doesn't hurt. It's not even more than a little bit uncomfortable. With the CT scan, you go into the clinic, get an IV of some kind of tracer compound and then go get the scan. They lay you on a table and sometimes pull a strap around you that holds your hands on your abdomen or chest. This strap is for comfort and keeps you from having to hold your arms and hands in a certain position for a period of time. Sometimes you will have to hold your arms stretched out over your head which is rather uncomfortable but it doesn't last long. The experience is different for each of us.

The table moves you into a tube-like apparatus which contains the camera that is taking pictures of whatever is going on inside your body. It's a lonely process but you may rest assured that you are being closely watched on a television screen nearby.

This is when you use the mantra:

"Everything is going to be all right."

The PET scans are a bit more complicated and they take more time. With the PET scan you need to go at least 6 hours without eating or drinking anything besides water. It took me a while to understand what was going on in the process. An hour or so before the scan the technician will check your blood for sugar level. Then she will install a port in your arm through which they will first put saline solution and then follow it up with a glucose solution. Then comes the easy part; you get to sit under a nice warm blanket in a recliner and read or nap while the glucose goes through your blood stream. The glucose is what somehow marks the suspected cancerous areas. The PET machine is larger than the CT scanner but similar in design and function. It takes seven three-minute pictures of parts of your body. These will be put together for the diagnosis. The total scan takes about 25 minutes.

I have developed the ability to lie very still, close my eyes, and let my mind roam wherever it wants to go. Anytime I feel any claustrophobia or other anxiety, I use the mantra.

"Everything is going to be all right."

I've talked with several people about the scans. The major problem with the scan process for some people seems to be claustrophobia—a fear of tight closed places. The medical staff can give you a pill for that or you can meditate your way out of it. I prefer the meditation process.

I lie on a long table on my back, hands and arms resting on my abdomen, staring at the ceiling. The table moves in and out, moving into the scanning circle and back out, always stopping at different places. The machine is calibrating itself. After a few minutes of this calibration the machine takes a short break.

The machine stops its in and out process and the table moves you into the circle, stopping in a position just at the end of the apparatus. You can get a glimpse of the ceiling and there is a sign on the machine itself that says, "Do not stare at the laser." Give me a break. If you don't want me to stare at something, hide it or at least don't tell me about it. After I read the little sign that said not to stare at the laser, it was all I could do to keep my eyes off it! So I stared at the ceiling. A gaggle of cardboard butterflies hung on strings, moving about in the wind of the air conditioner.

The table moves me back into position. A spinning noise comes out of the circle that surrounds my body. I concentrate on not staring at the laser which never comes on anyway. The spinning sound stops after a little while and the table moves me slightly to line me up for another segment of the picture taking process. At this point, I have figured out that I have seen all of the different motions I am going to see. I close my eyes and concentrate on clearing out all wayward thoughts by picturing a valley with a stream running through it as seen from a mountain top. My strategy works and my anxiety is lessened.

After I figure out the motions of the machine for the first of the seven scans, the rest of the process is easy to absorb and accept. I move my mind to the beautiful valley that I have created as a refuge and the machine takes six more three-minute pictures. The technician comes in, mutters some pleasantries, and helps me sit up. No problem.

And that's it. The scan results go to yet another specialist for analysis. There probably won't be another one for a few months. I also know that when another scan comes along, it won't be a new experience and I will know what to expect and how to handle it. Piece of cake.

"Everything is going to be all right."

The ultrasound as I understand it, is the same as the one used on a pregnant woman. I've never been pregnant so I wasn't familiar with it. All the ultrasound consists of is someone rubbing a flat thing all over the area of the suspected tumor and watching for it on television. Tumors (solid) will show up as white masses on the screen. Cysts (fluid filled) show up as black masses. Sound waves are sent into the body and bounce off things of different mass in different ways. Sometimes they will use this process to find out where to stick a needle and obtain tissue for a biopsy. Not to worry, though. Ultrasounds are painless.

FROM THE JOURNAL

They have to calibrate where the radiation will go so they scan you and then they mark a reference point for the radiation technicians to line you up properly.

The girl who was "calibrating" me asked, "Would you mind if we put a very small tattoo on your chest? That way it won't wash off."

I replied, "As long as it's a dragon tattoo."

She giggled, "All right, but you and I will be the only ones who know what it is. It will be too small for everyone else to see."

So now I know that I have a dragon tattoo on my chest but I'm damned if I can find it. When the lady said "small" that's what she meant.

From Sylvia

I was not allowed to read because my eye movement could throw off the test results since my cancer was in my head. Each patient is different.

I kept my eyes closed at all times during CT and PET scans. This kept claustrophobia at bay. I lay down on the table and never even looked at the machines.

"For myself I am an optimist—it does not seem to be much use to be anything else."

>**Winston Churchill**

"Nobody can take away the last of the human freedoms, which is one's ability to choose his or her attitude in any given set of circumstances."

>**Viktor Frankl**

CHAPTER 5

The Diagnosis and Treatment Plan

From a cancer specialist in 1850: "There are three ways to get rid of cancer. You can cut it out, you can burn it out, and you can poison it out."

Those words were written a long time ago. In 1850, doctors used lye to burn cancer out and arsenic to poison it out. We are much more sophisticated in the twenty first century, but the basic principles are the same.

The cancer center I attended has what is known as a "Tumor Board" which consists of several specialists who will study your particular problem and come up with a treatment plan. I would assume that all cancer centers have a Tumor Board by one name or another. The main idea of cancer treatment, as I understand it, is to kill the cancer cells and the other cells around that area. The cancer cells will not regenerate but the normal cells will.

My statement is probably overly simplistic from a clinical aspect, but it suits my purposes. The goal with this book is to throw out the simple information and open up a set of questions with which the reader may research at any level he or she desires.

At any rate, the Tumor Board has a multitude of options to consider for the treatment. It does seem to me, though, that most of the treatment options do revolve around the idea of "cut it out, burn it out, poison it out."

There is no point in my going into the myriad of treatment possibilities available to the members of the Tumor Board. I'm not qualified and that is also not within the intended scope of this book. I am just here to tell you that the possibilities of effective treatments being available are in your favor.

Some other types of cancer treatments:

—Targeted therapy

—Immunotherapy

—Hyperthermia

—Stem Cell Transplant (Peripheral Blood, Bone Marrow, and Cord Blood Transplants)

—Photodynamic therapy

I personally prefer "cut it out" when possible. My sister felt the same way and didn't hesitate to undergo a double mastectomy to get the offending cells removed. In my case, my larynx (voice box) was cut out and a tumor was surgically removed from my carotid artery. My only problem was that about six months later a couple of tumors reappeared on my shoulder around the artery and they were just too close to remove surgically. Following that episode, the Tumor Board recommended both radiation and chemotherapy.

Out of all of the possibilities available, your treatment plan will be carefully tailored to your needs. It is rather frightening when the oncologist presents you with the treatment plan. There will be all sorts of questions that need to be asked, but you really don't know what those questions are at that point. This means it is time for the mantra:

"Everything is going to be all right."

Sometimes the tumor has grown or spread to the point that it is not possible to cut it out and have a good chance of getting it all. Or the tumor may be located in a place inaccessible to surgery. My friend Sylvia's cancer was behind her eye, which meant that there was no way to cut it out, so it would have to be treated with radiation and chemo only.

FROM THE JOURNAL

Logging the new cancer treatment.
February 2013
Copy of family letter: written Feb 2, It took me a while to work on my discipline and write it but I knew it had to happen.

> *We were in the facilities at Emory from 2:00 until about 6:30 Friday. Radiation consultation with Dr. Higgins and chemo consultation with Dr. Saba. I am pleased with both of them . I had wanted to get the treatments moved to the clinic in Rome and avoid all of the traveling but since my surgery had been performed at Emory, the surgeon and her staff preferred*

that I use the facilities at Emory. Oh, well, lots of miles.

The thing on my shoulder is bigger and the chemo doctor said that the activity is "aggressive" They are going to hit it with all they got.

This is good news and bad news. Good news is that they are on it and going after it hard. Bad news is that I am expected to have a rough time of it.

The treatments will more than likely begin on the 12th of February. Everything will end up somewhere around the end of March. I have been fitted for the mask that holds me in the right place for the radiation. The radiation treatments don't take but 15–20 minutes and they will be given 5 days a week for 7 weeks. There will be three chemo treatments—Feb. 12, March 5, and March 26. All dates are approximate.

(The above was the original chemo plan. After a hearing test which showed hearing loss, the doctors determined that the original treatment may negatively affect my hearing and the treatments were changed to weekly ones of a different set of chemicals.)

The treatments will probably fry my neck a bit more severely than the previous radiation did and so they will install a feeding tube in my stomach to be used later on—I would suspect somewhere after the third or fourth week. The tube installation will be an overnight stay in the hospital.

As for the chemo, there are only six treatments but it takes several hours to administer each of them. They said that I can take a break during the infusion to go get a radiation treatment. Whee!! One of the possible side effects is hearing problems so I will have to have a hearing exam and profile so they will have a reference point in case something does go wrong.

All of that said, I am still of the belief that I will be getting the best treatment possible. I am greatly impressed with the situation at Emory. Get this, they even pay for valet parking just for me.

As I said, I should be finished with the treatments by April first. It will take some time to recover from the physical effects of the treatments, but I know all this by now. A few months after the treatments are over with I will have a PET scan to make sure that all is well.

The thing is, right now I feel very good and other than a little lump on my shoulder I wouldn't ever think there was anything wrong with me. I am therefore

35

most happy that the situation has been diagnosed and is being acted upon at this point.

Dekie is my leaning post and I don't know how I could handle things without her. Everyone wants to know what they can do to help and here's my reaction—If you notice that Dekie needs a leaning post, please offer her one.

Ok, that's done,
john

I guess that takes care of stating the problem and schedule. Dekie cried the first night we were back from the doctors...That Friday night when neither of us slept well. She's back to being her laughing self and I'm doing my thing about figuring out where the money is coming from.

Looking back, then, on the notes that I had written, it is easy to see just where my fears were coming from. I don't think I was as much afraid of the cancer or of croaking as I was apprehensive about the treatments themselves. I feel like this was a healthy attitude.

Curry Roasted Butternut Squash & Chickpeas

1 butternut squash, peeled, seeded, and cubed
1 sweet potato, peeled and cubed
1 can chickpeas, drained and rinsed
¼ c. olive oil
1 T. curry powder
3 T. honey
¼ t. cayenne pepper
orange juice, water

Preheat oven to 375°. In large bowl, mix vegetables with olive oil, curry powder, honey, cayenne pepper, and salt to taste. Spread onto a baking sheet in a single layer. Add orange juice and water to pan, and roast, turning occasionally, for about an hour, until vegetables are tender. Adjust seasonings if needed.

"Optimism is a strategy for making a better future. Because unless you believe that the future can be better, you are unlikely to step up and take responsibility for making it so."

➤**Noam Chomsky**

CHAPTER 6

Surgery: Cut It Out

Cut it out.

This is certainly the most straightforward method for removing the cancerous cells. The only problem is that surgery doesn't work a lot of the time. Sometimes it takes a combination of treatments to remove all of the cancerous growth.

By the time Dr. Chen got to me, I had a pretty bad tumor on my vocal cords and another wrapped halfway around my carotid artery. I knew I was in trouble and I knew I would have to have a laryngectomy which is the removal of the vocal cords. I was good with all of that and I had been told that my doctor was one of the best around.

An experience that sticks in my mind happened a couple of days before the operation when Dr. Chen said, "I'm going to go after the tumor on the carotid artery first. Then, if I get that, I will do the laryngectomy." I asked her why and she said, "If I can't get the tumor off the artery, I'll just sew you back up because there will be no reason to go any further."

I looked at her, alarmed. "And if that happens?" I asked.

She quietly replied, "Then you will die."

I think that's one of the most frightening things I ever

heard. I had to live with that knowledge for several days until it was time for the operation. That was a difficult time for me. Because of the tumor in my esophagus, I sometimes had a hard time breathing. I can vividly remember one time I was driving and had to pull off the road, get out of the truck, and practice some breathing exercises that I had learned from my tai chi teacher who also happens to be my wife. I can remember, at that point, looking forward to the operation.

Looking forward to having my vocal cords removed.

Looking forward to grasping for life and doing everything possible to hold on.

And I said to myself:

"Everything is going to be all right."

And I didn't really worry about dying. I was sure that everything would be all right. Optimism became the very best friend in my psychological arsenal.

On the designated morning we showed up at Emory at some ungodly hour in the morning. My orders were processed and Dekie and I sat and talked and held hands. Her parents joined us later. I know that my mother was beside herself in a far away town. Here I was undergoing serious surgery and my brother, Billy had just died a few short weeks before. The operation took seven or eight hours. I probably had it easier than anyone in the family during that time because I was in never-never land. I do remember waking up, though. It was as if someone had flipped a light switch. There I was looking up at family members and the doctor. I had one question—I looked straight at the doctor and asked silently, "Did you get it?"

She smiled brightly and said, "Yes."

I'll never forget how I felt when I heard that. It was euphoria brought on by total relief. I realized that when I asked the question there was no sound because she had removed my voice box. I also realized that she knew exactly what I had been asking.

After the surgery, cancer really ceased to be a problem as I used all of my energy recuperating and learning how to cope with not being able to speak. I used a pen and paper to communicate. A sweet young speech therapist brought me an "electrolarynx" and tried her best to get me to practice with it. I tried for a bit but I just couldn't get the hang of it. I have always been a highly verbal person and I have had pride in my well-developed vocabulary. The electrolarynx was apparently too limiting for me and I subconsciously rejected it in favor of writing—which I could do well.

The speech therapist obviously ratted me out to a couple of the doctors, because early one morning they gave me a hard time about being un-cooperative regarding the electrolarnyx. I still don't think I was out of line. I just think that I was coping with the situation the best I could. I think perhaps my mind was rebelling against the possibility of failure. I would not fail with writing. I knew that.

I think the point I am making is that we should deal with the psychology of healing on our own terms. This is not to say we should not ask for help but that we should be allowed to evaluate the help and use it as we see fit.

Thinking deeper into the subject, I would assume that

with a lot of surgeries there is a sense of loss. I lost my larnyx. A mastectomey patient loses her breasts. Both can be important, life changing losses. I'm sure there are many more situations in which the sense of loss would occur. If this happens to you and you need help, ask. It will be there for you. It is all right to grieve through the sense of loss, but one should watch carefully for signs of depression if the grief becomes overwhelming or lasts for an extended period of time.

I am sometimes saddened when I think about the fact that I will never again be able to play the guitar and sing along, but then I work that around in my mind and realize that it is just a trade off for LIFE. Losing my voice box is a trade off for being able to spend more time with my wonderful wife, family, and friends. I get to watch the sun rise and walk in the snow with Ziplock baggies on my feet. I get to read in bed or write poetry. Now, I can smile and listen to John Denver singing about Tools the baby rabbit and I can sing along in my mind while I play the air guitar. Dekie says that I will be all the way back when I pick up the guitar and play it with no expectations of being able to sing.

A year and a half after the life-saving operation, I was blessed with a granddaughter. At this writing, Margot is six months old and she always grins when I talk to her with my funny voice. I'm glad I got to live for that.

Your surgery may or may not be as life changing as mine was or it may be much more drastic than I could ever imagine. At any rate, whatever you have lost, think of it as a trade-out instead of a loss. You have traded for *life.*

42

In my case the surgery was successful and I was alive and learning to live without a voice. A five month period spent communicating with a notepad taught me quite a lot about other people's limitations. I was eventually fitted with a prosthesis that allows me to talk by using the muscles in my throat that are normally used for burping. It's an amazingly simple device that works well. It takes time but at the writing of this I am now gaining expertise and confidence with the device. I am now considering public speaking as an option.

An excerpt from my journal turned into a reading for the Rome Area Writers. I tried to do it with the electro-larynx but it didn't work and I had to get someone else to read it for me:

FROM THE JOURNAL

October, 2012
The nicest thing about the operation is that I can breathe again.
Breathing is under-rated and taken for granted until...
Until it becomes difficult or impossible to breathe.
Then we notice...Oh, yeah, then we notice.

A doctor in an emergency room once told me, "Blood goes round and round, air goes in and out. Any deviation from this is not good." I found this statement funny and quotable until the day I had to

43

pull the truck over to the curb and get out to do some deep breathing exercises just to keep from passing out. That's when the doctor's statement rang true.

I have learned a lot about the larynx (or voice box) over the last two or three years. I have a feeling that I am going to learn a lot more. In case you have forgotten since your high school science class, I'll refresh you: there are two pipes going down your throat—the esophagus for food and liquids and the trachea for air and sound. The back of the tongue is designed to cover the trachea when you swallow and dump all the swallowings down the proper pipe. One does not want foreign matter in the air pipe.

The larynx is the organic device that makes sound so that we can talk. Most of us know that. What a lot of us don't know is that the larynx is also the last gate before the lungs. If even a little bit of foreign matter reaches it to the larynx, we begin to cough until that matter is removed. Larger matter in the trachea causes us to choke and to die of asphyxiation. This is not pleasant.

Sometimes, due to cancer and/or other reasons, it is necessary to remove the voice box. This is called a laryngectomy. What they do is cut that sucker out and re-direct the air to a new hole in the neck. This is called a "stoma." I knew about stomas because they are also little things on the underside of a leaf that allow for oxygen transfer. Stomas are important.

I knew what was going to happen to me, but it still took some getting used to. I went to the hospital for an operation, got gassed, and woke up with a hole in my throat and no voice.

If you know me at all, you know that I'm always open for an adventure. You know that I am interested in new knowledge gained from new experiences. And you know that I am a true optimist. If you don't know me, then please just take my word for it. At any rate I was ready to learn all about my new adventure.

You see, the laryngectomy operation re-directs the air and it doesn't move in or out through the mouth any more. I never knew that air through my mouth did so many things. I'm learning. Did you realize that when you take a sip of water, you actually draw it in with air? I didn't know that until after the operation when I found that I had to drink in a slightly different manner. What about blowing on a spoon full of soup to cool it off before putting it in your mouth? No more of that, either. I burned my tongue three times before learning.

I can't blow my nose or spit. No more whistling. I always wanted to go squirrel hunting with an Indian blow gun—that ain't going to happen, either. The squirrels are safe—but then, they were probably safe before the operation, too. One day I tried to gargle with mouthwash—nope, that didn't work. I keep learning about new things that I can't do.

But what I CAN do is **breathe**. I sure do like being able to breathe again and I feel so much better. Breathing is good.

I haven't really tried it yet, but I'll bet I can set a new record for kissing because I can do that and breathe at the same time. I won't have to come up for air.

As I write this, three weeks after the operation, my throat is still swollen from the stitches that were necessary to keep my esophagus from leaking. A leaking esophagus is not good. I had to be fed through a nasal tube and was told that I was not to swallow for fourteen days after the operation. The not swallowing was a difficult assignment. I was very happy the day the tube came out.

I am now waiting for the swelling in my throat to go away so that I can see about getting a new store bought voice box. In the mean time, if I want to converse with someone, I use either the electrolarynx or my notebook and pen. I find interactions with people to be fun, interesting, and sometimes frustrating. I know that not being able to talk is a short range thing for me, but the people I am trying to converse with don't realize this.

Reactions to the electrolarynx are varied. Most people are not familiar with the purpose of the device and, therefore, are wary of even trying to understand or relate to what is going on as I use it. The therapist told me it takes practice. I have done that and I feel like I've made progress in the use of the device. The therapist told me that the success of the device also depends on the participation of the person with whom I am communicating. A lot of people don't understand this part.

Writing as a form of communication is fun, also — especially when I mistakenly assume that the other person can read.

A number of people look at my writing and my smile and assume that I am also hearing impaired. That's when they start making hand motions and moving their lips in an effort to be helpful. When that happens, I write on my tablet in large letters — I CAN HEAR. They usually don't pay attention to that, though. They just go on moving their hands around and shouting.

One day soon I will be able to talk **and** breathe. I am looking forward to that.

"Be of good cheer. Do not think of today's failures, but of the success that may come tomorrow. You have set yourselves a difficult task, but you will succeed if you persevere; and you will find a joy in overcoming obstacles. Remember, no effort that we make to attain something beautiful is ever lost."

➤**Helen Keller**

CHAPTER 7

Radiation: Burn It Out

Burn it out.

It is my opinion that radiation is the easiest of the cancer treatments to tolerate even though the after-effects can be severe.

The actual radiation treatment consists of the patient reclining on a table and a machine shooting a radiation beam into the cancerous area of the body. Since the process involves daily treatments over a six week period (more or less), some method for easily and accurately lining the patient's body up with the ray gun must be worked out.

I found the set-up process for radiation treatments most interesting because it is so precise. As I understand it the idea is to aim the radiation in such a manner that it burns only the cancer cells and a small area around them.

A CT scan is made to find the exact area of the body that the ray gun will treat. The technicians will mark the area with magic markers or some sort of tape or marker that gives a reference point. In one case, I received a small tattoo. I know it was there because they told me it was but I never saw it. It must have been tiny.

The next step is to devise some sort of a mask or other type of device that will hold your body in place while the treatment is being administered. Since my cancer was in my throat, my device had to hold my head perfectly still in a certain position. The technicians made a custom-fitted mask that bolted me down to the table. Each time I entered the treatment room, I glanced at a wall on my left. There hung a multitude of molded devices to accommodate each of the patients undergoing treatments at that time. Each patient had his or her own personal hook-up to be used for lining them up to the machine.

My first radiation treatment was rather tense because of the natural tendency of a human to fear the unknown. I was ready for whatever happened, though, and the people who work in the radiation center are very kind and try their best to make you feel comfortable and easy with the process. I also repeated my mantra to give myself confidence.

"Everything is going to be all right."

I felt a bit of claustrophobia as I was fastened to the table. The technician made some adjustments and walked out of the room. The lights were low but I could see that someone had taken time to hang some cardboard butterflies from the ceiling. I lay there motionless and after a few minutes the machine started humming and moving around above my head. I never did figure out quite what was happening but there was no pain or other sensation. I think at times throughout the treatments I felt some small tingling sensation but it may have just been an illusion. Other than being pinned down to a table, the experience was not unpleasant.

Even though there was no actual sensation at the time of the treatments, as time went by the effects of the radiation started showing up. At first it was like a mild sunburn on the outside and then it progressed to a more severe burn. As time went by the radiation on my throat caused it to swell and it became harder for me to swallow. I could feel a burning inside and a bit of pain if I ate the wrong things. I started a soup diet. They had installed a feeding tube in my stomach, but I was too stubborn to use it.

One of the wonderful ideas that I was living with throughout the radiation treatment for tumors on my carotid artery was that the doctor had told me, "There is an eight percent chance that your carotid artery will explode and you will die."

I thought about it and the prospect didn't sound at all pleasant. I asked the doctor, "What will it feel like if it explodes?"

She replied, "You won't feel it. It will be that fast."

One of the things I like to do with thoughts like that is to stick them in the back of my mind and pretend they don't exist. I buried the exploding artery idea deep down inside most rapidly.

It doesn't take long to get used to the radiation treatments and they just become a daily chore. You go to the treatment center, wait your turn, get fastened to the table, get zapped, and leave. One of the side effects of the radiation treatments is fatigue but I believe that a lot of the fatigue is from the drudgery of going for the treatments day after day after day.

When I started the treatments I could actually feel the

tumors on my shoulder. I checked them daily and about halfway through my treatments, I could detect a notable decrease in size. This made me very happy and I often found myself reaching up to check the tumors and grinning as they slowly became smaller.

So all in all, taking radiation treatments is normally not all that big a thing. I know that some treatment regimens are more difficult than others due to where and how far advanced the cancer is. The chemo is the treatment that makes you really feel bad and makes your hair fall out.

You know, I kept waiting for that carotid artery to explode. I also kept feeling the two knots on my shoulder that were the tumors. The chemo made me feel bad. The radiation made me feel tired. The three hours a day of driving five days a week made me feel like I was in a tunnel. Feeling the knots on my shoulder every day and noticing that they were getting softer and smaller made me feel wonderful. It was getting easier and easier for me to say,

"Everything is going to be all right."

There's something about finding that one thing that makes you feel good and then focusing your energies on it. I decided that I wouldn't think much about the other things. I just concentrated on the good part. I enjoyed knowing that my discomfort was moving the problem in a positive direction.

That's optimism. Optimism can be learned. With practice, optimism will become easier and better. It will grow and prosper, so to speak. Look on the bright side. One of the figures I ran across in my reading was that there are 14 million people living in the United States who either have, or have had, cancer. You are not alone by any means.

FROM THE JOURNAL (I take lessons on being judgmental)

I usually have to wait ten minutes, more or less, for my radiation treatment. I've had a little banter with a number of people who wait with me.

The coffee machine in the waiting room is awesome.

One guy comes with his wife to drive him and he has the nastiest attitude. I told Sweetie about it. She said maybe something was wrong in his life.

I said, "Maybe things are not going within the scope of his plans."

She replied, "Well, everyone should have dealing with cancer in their plans. It just seems to affect so many people."

I found out later that the man had been having a rather hard time with his chemo treatments that he was taking simultaneously with the radiation.

I guess it never pays to be judgmental until you know the rest of the story.

"I meant to write about death, only life came breaking in as usual"

➤Virginia Woolf

"Happiness is a butterfly, which when pursued, is always just beyond your grasp, but which, if you will sit down quietly, may alight upon you."

➤Nathaniel Hawthorne

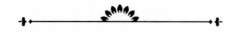

CHAPTER 8

Chemotherapy: Poison It Out

FROM THE JOURNAL, February 2013

In adversity, look to the little things and enjoy them.
The chemo took away most of my sense of taste
But it left me coffee. I appreciated that.
It was cold in the chemo infusion room
But they gave me a pre-warmed blanket when I entered.
It was cold and bleak in late winter
But when I looked closely,
The growth buds on the trees were swelling and about to open.
I felt old and ill and ugly
And then I got a hug from someone who said,
"Everything is going to be all right."
And it was.

Poison it out.

They refer to it as "chemo." This is one of the areas in which new treatments are constantly being developed. This is also the cancer treatment with the side effects that we relate to "having cancer."

From what I understand (and please remember that I was an English major in college) cancer cells grow faster than healthy cells, crowding them out. Therefore, the chemicals used in chemo treatments are developed to kill fast-growing cells. Some parts of our bodies also consist of quickly growing cells, even in healthy situations. Examples are hair, fingernails, and taste buds. Because these normal healthy cells are fast growers, the chemotherapy medications target them as well as cancerous growth. This is why a lot of people lose their hair during treatment.

As with the radiation, the chemo oncologist will prescribe a certain number of treatments (or "infusions"). Sometimes treatments with pills may be used. Also as in radiation, a finite number of treatments will be prescribed.

As with radiation, you can mark on your calendar when the treatments will occur. After every treatment, make a big X over the square on the calendar. Next to that write "6 MORE" (or whatever the number is). This will give you a countdown chart. This will give you something to rejoice over and the effects of the rejoicing will help to carry you through. Any time you get depressed during the treatments, you can look at the calendar and say,

"Everything is going to be all right."

Due to the uncertainty of the effects, you will probably need a driver on chemo days. During my treatments I could handle driving most of the time but when asked about my transportation arrangements, I would always smile and say, "Sweetie drives on chemo days."

If you don't have a sweetie or a friend to drive, talk to the people at the cancer clinic. They are wonderful about working out problems. There are also many programs around to give or find any assistance you require during your treatments.

There are lots of blood tests involved with chemo. I think that usually you will get a test before each treatment to check your white blood cell count and other things I don't know much about.

A large percentage of chemo patients are fitted with a "port." This is a semi-permanent implant that makes it easier to administer the infusion. The port is pretty gross and unpleasant to think about, but once it's in, there's no big deal and it makes the process so much easier in that the technicians don't have to find a vein to insert a needle for every treatment. I've had a port before. It was in my shoulder. I just laughed and referred to it as my "grease fitting."

The process of the chemical infusion was not all that unpleasant as far as I was concerned. It was the same as getting any other sort of IV injection. I lay back in a special recliner (o.k. it *was* a little bit short for my six foot two inch frame) and the nurses ran a tube into my arm from a bag hanging on a rack. The rack had wheels on it in case I needed to go to the bathroom. They gave me a Benadryl injection before the chemo and by the time I was receiving the chemo meds by IV, I really didn't worry about much. I had my ubiquitous book, there were plenty of televisions, snack carts rolled through occasionally, and I pretty much succumbed to the Benadryl and slept.

I remember once, in the middle of my Benadryl-induced sleep, I was awakened by a nutritionist who wanted to get all kinds of information from me. This was right after I had just gotten my artificial voice and she couldn't seem to understand me. (this was probably because I was half asleep). I resorted to writing the answers longhand on a piece of paper and the lady soon gave up on the interview. I found the notes later and realized why—the writing was totally unreadable. It was tiny and cramped. Funny, it seemed so clear at the time.

FROM THE JOURNAL:

I thought this set of notes was funny. I am including it unedited and straight from the iPhone:

4

Chemo

2/13

Fancy coffee in the main lobby. No phone signal. Rules and regs.

One funny thing—all the nurses check out my veins first thing. Today I jokingly said "I shall try to furnish you with a decent vein." She pointed at my arm and informed me that she had already picked one out.

Pharmacist just informed us they changed the meds on account of my hearing. This means once a week treatments.

They injected me with Benadryl for allergies.

They can't find scrips from the other day so they're calling in more.

Getting sleepy.

11:13. Hooking me up. Checked and double che

As you can see, the Benadryl kicked in right in the middle of a word. Other than having a needle stuck in your arm, it's not a totally unpleasant experience. My personal chemo schedule was on a weekly basis. My wife, Dekie, would drive me to the clinic and make sure all was well. She would then go for a walk or visit friends until my treatment was finished. I really didn't want her to have to sit there and wait all day.

Dekie and I were impressed with the sheer number of treatment bays that are available. There must have been close to a hundred at the Emory Clinic and they were kept full most of the time.

There is a bell fastened to a wall at the Emory Infusion Center that is to be rung only by patients completing their treatments. One of my nicest memories is ringing that bell and everyone in the clinic applauding. It brought tears to my eyes. I knew that we were all in it together. I wrote a story about that day.

One of the things I noticed about the chemo side effects was that I could never seem to get warm. The chemotherapy happened during a period that started the first of February and was finished around the end of the first week in April. The weather was getting better and better but I never felt warm. When I was home dealing with my personal version of "chemo brain" (a term for treatment-caused disorientation), I would dress as warmly as possible to keep from having to turn the thermostat way up and make Dekie uncomfortable. This worked pretty well but my fingers remained cold. A number of people going through the treatments, along with a number of cancer veterans, told me that the same thing had been true with them.

I enjoyed the fact that every time I went into the clinic for my process they had a pre-warmed blanket for me to use. When I started out with the treatments I noticed several ladies wearing toboggans and I thought this was to cover up for a loss of hair. I very quickly figured out that they were just trying to keep their ears warm. I never cease to be amazed with how rapidly one's perceptions can change when given a bit of additional information.

FROM THE JOURNAL

Progress report,
Sunday, March 17

Friday visit with the chemo doctor was uneventful. I've decided that being a chemo doctor must be the cushiest job in the world. He asks a few questions, makes a few comments, looks in my mouth, and nods to the nurse. He gets a good pay rate, too. I bet there are some princes and kings that ain't got it so good.

Anyway, I seem to be doing better than any chemo patient in the history of the world or something like that. It is starting to show, though. No taste for anything and due to the effects of the radiation on my throat, I have to drink my meals. I have cans of calories and I need to drink 3 or 4 of them a day. I use a steady rinse of saltwater with baking soda all day to help with the damages from the radiation and chemo in my mouth. Even ice cream has no taste or appeal and if you know about my special relationship with ice cream, you can appreciate the devastation of this development. I still halfway enjoy my coffee, though, so all is not lost. It's kind of funny that at a time I can have anything I want—I don't want anything. (I just re-read that last statement and realized the true humor in it.)

I now have only twelve more visits to Atlanta for the extent of the treatment schedule. Two of those visits will involve radiation and chemo infusion, the other ten are for just radiation. The chemo will be on the 20th and 27th and then will be no more. (It will take several weeks for the chemo effects to wear off so I don't know when I will take Joel Todino up on the two inch thick prime filet that he is saving for me.)

Michener, in his book Alaska, wrote about the phenomenon of suicides increasing right before the end of the long nights. An observer remarked, "But they only had a couple of more weeks to go." The narrator replied, "Yes, but they just couldn't take it any longer." This is important to me as it helps me to realize that the hardship of waiting for the end intensifies as things get nearer to the end. I am observing less motivation in myself at the moment. I just don't want to do much of anything but yet I'm bored. Does that make sense?

The swelling in my throat from the radiation makes talking a bit more difficult but I'm happy that I am able to talk anyway. I'm betting that after the radiation effects go away—probably about the end of April—I will be able to hone the talking into something rather nice. I'm bonding with my voice prosthesis more and more every day. Funny how a piece of plastic pipe can gain such importance.

So, onward for next week. I will start with Bob and Micheline driving me for the treatments on Monday, Dekie will drive on chemo day, and my friend Bud will pick up the last of the week. If you remember, Bud was a hero in Requiem for a Redneck. He keeps me laughing.

I am writing from the delightful glassed-in front porch at here at home. It is a wonderful sunny day and I am watching the robins, chipmunks, squirrels as they watch the women walking their dogs. Quite the entertainment. I think I will spend the day here *and ponder.*

I get tickled when I read back over that set of notes and see where I thought it would only take a few weeks for the effects of the chemo to go away. I'm writing this more than a year and a half later and I can still feel the effects. My sense of taste is just now starting to return. My fingers are still cold and Sweetie and I are still having a thermostat war. The ulcers in my mouth have gone away, though.

I think the thing I miss most is taste and I am encouraged with each change for the better, no matter how small. I have learned a most interesting thing about a drink named LaCroix. At one time in my life I had a problem with alcohol. One day I realized that it was ruining my life and on Thanksgiving day in the year 2001, I quit. I remember it well; it was 8:00 in the morning and I had a conversation with a beer can and threw it into the woods. I never drank alcohol again and my life immediately began to get a lot better. That's the background.

One of the problems with being what they call a "reforming alcoholic" is that you are used to always having a drink in your hand. This was definitely a problem for me. I tried a lot of different beverages and settled on coffee. One day after a year or so, a friend who was in the process of quitting drinking introduced me to LaCroix, which is a flavored, non-sweetened carbonated water. I thought it was one of the most God-awful tasting drinks ever and stuck to my coffee. I enjoyed herbal tea in the evenings after caffeine started interfering with my sleep.

Fast forward a few years. I started radiation and chemo

for throat cancer. I still liked my coffee, but it dried my mouth out too much after a few cups. Tea had lost its taste. I tried LaCroix again. It tasted wonderful! Actually, at the time it was, and now remains, one of the few drinks I can taste at all. I found it strange but interesting that I could only taste the lime flavored version—the other flavors didn't work.

I found that whenever I went to a restaurant, LaCroix was never available, so I would order a glass of water without ice, and a cup of coffee. I was having trouble finding suitable food at restaurants anyway, but I was trying to normalize my life and my wonderful wife tried so hard to cook good food for me that I wanted her to be able to occasionally eat at a restaurant. I really just wanted my special drink. That would make me happy.

Then I figured it out—I'm a cancer survivor, I can do anything I please! I therefore decided to just put a can of LaCroix in my jacket pocket and take it in with me. I had decided that if anyone said anything about my beverage, I would offer to pay for an empty glass. Of course, when I punch the button in my throat to talk, it is immediately apparent to the server that I have experienced some trauma. I was tickled to find out that the waitress would merely glance at my canned beverage and immediately ask me if I would like to have a glass. (I always have to specify "no ice"). Problem solved, and I learned a lesson.

From Sylvia

With an infusion every 3 weeks the first week you feel fine, the second week you crash, and the third week you bounce back only to be hit again.

Knit caps should be worn at night to keep the bald head warm.

Room temperature water is easier for chemo patients to drink—plus it helps to keep the body temp from dropping any lower.

Write it on your heart
that every day is the best day in the year.
He is rich who owns the day, and no one owns the day
who allows it to be invaded with fret and anxiety

Finish every day and be done with it.
You have done what you could.
Some blunders and absurdities, no doubt crept in.
Forget them as soon as you can, tomorrow is a new day;
begin it well and serenely, with too high a spirit
to be cumbered with your old nonsense.

This new day is too dear,
with its hopes and invitations,
to waste a moment on the yesterdays.

➤**Ralph Waldo Emerson**
Collected Poems and Translations

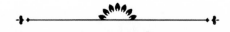

CHAPTER 9

The Waiting Room and the Regimen

I call it "The Regimen." I guess it could also be called "The Mission." The Regimen consists of showing up for a radiation treatment five days a week for six weeks, more or less, according to your circumstances. It's not that the treatment hurts, or that it takes all that much time. The main thing about The Regimen is that one must work the day around it—every day.

The radiation techs are dealing with a lot of people every day and they run a tight schedule. Other than times when there was a technical problem or an equipment breakdown, I never had to wait much more than ten or fifteen minutes at the most. The treatment then takes ten or fifteen minutes. At first, just the thought of going through the radiation regimen is intimidating but after a few sessions the experience becomes routine and mundane. The radiation techs and schedulers are more than happy to work around the patient's time preferences. Most employers, too, seem to be willing to help arrange a time that is convenient for clinic visits. Everyone involved should just realize that the radiation process only lasts for a prescribed number of weeks and then it will be over with.

I am an early riser, and I found that it was relatively easy to get my visits scheduled between seven and seven thirty in the mornings. I realized that a lot of people don't like to get up and out early and I turned that fact to my advantage. I could show up, have a cup of coffee in the waiting room, speak to a few nice people, get zapped, and then resume the activities of the day. The regimen became comfortable and almost enjoyable. I began to look forward to the treatments themselves as an enforced opportunity for meditation.

I found the first two or three radiation visits to be a bit stressful because I didn't know what to expect. I soon understood what was going on, however, and decided to deal with the stress and fear by concentrating on a short period of meditation. The techs would arrange my body on the machine's table, start the process, and then leave the room to avoid the radiation. At that point, I learned to throw my mind out of gear—to shift into neutral, so to speak—and to move into another world. Sometimes I would travel in my mind to a peaceful lake and watch the butterflies. Other times I would recline on a quiet mountain-top and study the clouds. This period of meditation gave me a feeling of peace and well-being, making the treatments short and pleasant. I made good use of the mantra:

"Everything is going to be all right."

The radiation waiting room can be sad and somber or it can be very interesting. A lot of the time the nature of the experience will depend on you. All of the people waiting are there for the same reason, more or less, but they're on a different schedule. Some patients are just starting and are not sure what to expect. Others are "old veterans" and are almost finished. Some feel good, some are tired, and some feel very bad from chemo treatments that they get on the side. I had a number of fun conversations—some of which I instigated and others that just happened.

FROM THE JOURNAL:

I got to talking to a guy from Newnan in the waiting room. I am half way through my treatments and he is just starting. He said he had a brain tumor that was still at the treatable stage.

I asked him how he felt about it.

"I'm a likker salesman," he said. "I've been doing it for twenty years and I make a really good living. I love my job and I love my family."

He paused, looked at the floor and looked back up at me, smiling.

"I never would have known about this tumor except that a lady ran a red light and ran into the side of my car. I hit my head. Just to make sure I was all right, the people at the emergency room did a scan. They found the tumor and here I am with a good chance of being cured."

He looked at me and shook his head.

"Ain't it funny? If that lady hadn't run that red light, the tumor would have been too big to treat in a few months.

"I sure am lucky."

I loved his attitude!

I shared this story with my friend Diana Smithson and I loved her response to it:

I, like you, met so many angels while waiting my turn in the radiation or chemo treatment waiting room. You would usually meet different folks going through what you were going through and you would sit and talk to each other like old friends while waiting your turn to go into treatment. Knowing you may not run into this person again, so you visited like old friends who had the same thing in common. In an odd way I miss that. Because while in treatment, as hard as it was on you, you knew you would run across someone that had the same thing in common with you and it always was an odd comfort to you, and you actually looked forward to having someone to talk to, someone that really understood what you were going through at that time. Now, 6 years in remission for me and my family, I have never felt so alone living with this knowledge of knowing how going through cancer has affected me. It is with you every day. Though you don't want to admit it, it is there. The man you wrote about has the attitude we can all attest to. I agree with you.

The observations and conversations in the waiting room also made me aware of many things that were going on around me. This newly gained knowledge heightens my understanding of some of the things that may be affecting those around me. The basis for the following story would not have occurred to me before my experiences in the radiation waiting room.

LEON

Leon was an outstanding carpet installer in his time
But that's not a job for an old guy.
So I often see him at work helping people
In his orange Home Depot apron.

I was a bit perturbed the other day
When a push buggy was blocking me
From being where I wanted to be
But I noticed that Leon was loading the buggy.

I smiled and pushed the button on my throat to speak
To Leon in my raspy voice.
Leon couldn't shake hands because he
Was holding a paint can in each hand

71

And loading the cart for a pretty lady.

When I spoke, she tured to look at me.
That happens to me a lot. But this time it was different
I turned my attention to her—
A pretty lady in a nice, full, long skirt—
And saw that she was completely bald.

But her eyes were what I really saw
They were large and dark as she looked at me.
Her eyes were weary and fear laden
Wordlessly, she looked into my eyes
And, wordlessly, I looked back into hers.

There was a silent exchange of feeling.
 I'm sure the look only lasted a moment
But it seemed like a very long time.
And I smiled a bit as I saw
Some of her fear subside.

Because, you see, we both realized in that instant
That I knew what she was going through
And that she knew where I had been.
Leon dropped a can of paint into the shopping cart
And I moved on to the plumbing department.

I wanted to say to her,
"Everything is going to be all right."

And maybe I did in one way or another.

Squash Casserole

3 lbs. yellow crookneck squash
½ onion, chopped
½ c. plain breadcrumbs
½ t. pepper
1 t. salt
Dash nutmeg
2 eggs, lightly beaten
¼ c. butter, divided.

Roughly chop the squash. Boil with the onion until very tender, approximately 10 minutes. Pour squash/onion mixture into colander and allow to drain very thoroughly. Gently mash mixture to squeeze out even more liquid. Transfer to a bowl, add ½ the butter, the bread crumbs, eggs and seasonings and mix well. Transfer to buttered casserole. Melt remaining butter and drizzle on top of squash. Bake at 350 for about 30 minutes, until lightly browned and bubbly.

"One of the things I learned the hard way was that it doesn't pay to get discouraged. Keeping busy and making optimism a way of life can restore your faith in yourself."

➤Lucille Ball

"My friends, love is better than anger. Hope is better than fear. Optimism is better than despair. So let us be loving, hopeful, and optimistic. We can change the world."

➤Jack Layton

CHAPTER 10

The Side Effects

As I stated earlier, the main side effects of radiation have to do with the "burning" nature of the treatment. These effects may range from a skin rash to a situation that resembles sunburn. Since the radiation penetrates the skin, there will be some burning and swelling underneath, also. This, of course, is the nature of the radiation treatment. I chuckled to myself when I related it to Superman's x-ray vision. The good thing about the radiation side effects (if there could be considered a good side) is that the radiation is limited to a localized area of the body.

Chemotherapy, on the other hand, due to its nature, will affect the entire body. There are many different chemicals that may be used for the chemo treatments and this fact, coupled with the inherent differences in each person's body, mean that there is no way to specifically predict how your particular body will react. I think because of this, the doctor's staff will only offer limited observations on what may happen. The patient is left to find out for herself.

Fatigue and nausea are the first and most prevalent symptoms to appear. I think these symptoms are rather short-lived and easy to deal with. The best way to deal with the fatigue is, of course, to rest and sleep. This resting is good for you anyway, and will help with the overall healing process. I'm sure that issuing a prescription for nausea medication is standard practice with beginning chemo patients.

After a few treatments, because of the fact that the chemo treatments kill quick-growing cells, hair often becomes affected. This occurrence may range from hair becoming thin and bodiless to just falling out. A lot of people view hair loss as a horror story but, you know what? It's going to come back again after the cancer is gone and you're going to live to see it. At least that's my attitude. Of course, there's always the mantra:

"Everything's going to be all right."

Other possible side effects are mouth ulcers and difficulty with swallowing. Saliva production may be affected, but there are pills to deal with this. All of these side effects are things that come and then will go away. To deal with them, we need the mantra:

"Everything's going to be all right."

The side effect of chemotherapy that I think is most significant—or it is in my case—is the loss of taste. Before I started the chemo treatments, a nurse practitioner told me to get plastic eating utensils and put the metal ones back in the drawer because the metal ones would impart a metallic taste to my food. I listened and did as I was told, but I found out that what the lady said did not happen to me. I have a funny story about how I found out that my sense of taste had been compromised:

It was on a Thursday. Dekie had taken me to Atlanta for my second chemo treatment on the previous day. I know it was a Thursday because the chemo treatments were always on Wednesday. Anyway, after Sweetie took me to my chemo session and back home, she left me to my own devices and went on a getaway trip with her father. We knew that the effects of the treatments would be cumulative and she wanted a break in case things got bad later on. I didn't blame her.

So, I was on my own for a few days. No problem. I was able to make the 5:00 a.m. trip to Atlanta for my radiation treatments and then to come home and attend to my job. She would only be gone for four days and two of the days would be weekend. No problem. Everything would be all right.

I remember it well. The first afternoon that I was alone, a Facebook friend mentioned that she had baked an apple pie for her husband. I pictured a steaming hot slice of pie with vanilla ice cream on top and immediately got in the truck and headed for the local Kroger store. I spent a bit of time studying the frozen pies and chose what looked like a good one. This would be my treat. One of the things about going through cancer treatments is that you can get any treat you want. I really wanted that pie.

It takes a long time to cook a frozen pie, too. It has to be thawed and baked just right. I followed the directions carefully. I cooked that pie just right. It was late when the pie got ready and I knew I should be in the bed to rest up for the following day, but I rubbed my hands together, smiled, and cut me a big slice. I put ice cream on top and just stood and admired the creation. Then I put some of it in my mouth.

It tasted terrible. I decided that I would take the pie back to the store the next day. There must be something wrong with it. I didn't take it back, though, I just threw it away a day or two later.

The next day I decided that it had been years since I had eaten a tuna and noodle casserole made with condensed cream of mushroom soup. This had always been one of my favorites. I remembered that my mother would make the casserole for me when I was sick. I had such good memories of that wonderful dish, so I cooked one up. I'll bet you have already guessed. It tasted terrible. I tried, but I just couldn't tolerate the taste. I punished myself mentally telling myself over and over, "I can't believe you messed up an easy recipe like that." The coonhound loved it, though.

Then the day after that, being a little slow and still not realizing that my sense of taste had been compromised by the chemo treatments, I decided to go to what I was really good at. I carefully put together a pot of my famous chili. I worked hard at it and simmered it slowly for hours before sitting down to eat a bowl of it. You guessed it. The taste of the chili was in between terrible and none at all. That's when I knew something was wrong with my sense of taste. The coonhound loved the chili.

That's the way it goes with chemo; the side effects sneak up on you and you have to figure out how to deal with them one at the time. The consolation is that in most cases the side effects will go away after the treatment. Some of them linger quite a while, though. The loss of taste is one of these. That's why the recipes are included in this book. These are some of the dishes that I know I liked during the chemo rounds.

Time for the mantra:

"Everything is going to be all right."

FROM THE JOURNAL

March 11 progress report
Doctor Higgins is becoming more and more pregnant. I hope she makes it to the end of my treatment. She and Ulrike, the nurse practitioner, checked me out today. They were amazed at my progress and at my lack of complications. Actually, Dr. Higgins said "You are amazing." I told her I preferred to be called "badass" so she called me that and laughed.

The inside of my mouth is doing well—not expected

The radiation burnt place is doing well—same

I was told that not being able to taste food was normal and was cautioned to have Dekie smell my food to make sure it warn't spoilt. The taste thing should last some weeks beyond the final chemo application. That will give me time to get my teeth fixed and then find the best steak in the world.

I was told that I have finished 19 radiation treatments

and have 16 more to go.

Wednesday will be my fifth of seven chemo treatments.

I'm feeling more and more tired but I'm able to function and that makes me happy.

So it's onward with the plan.

The tumor is diminishing in size—noticeably. It's pretty neat that I can see and feel it. It doesn't tingle any more, either.

A follow up on the above note is that it is now almost a year later and I still haven't eaten the steak. There are two reasons for this:

1. I have no taste for red meat any more which is pretty funny considering the fact that red meat was always one of my most favorite foods.

2. I have trouble swallowing stringy meats.

The upside of this is that I am enjoying soups and vegetables more than ever before. I'm sure that this is better for me, also.

FROM THE JOURNAL

I got my dentures fixed and then got a couple of horrible and painful mouth ulcers. Dr. Hortman, the dentist, worked on the appliance and told me to come back if things didn't get better. It took me a couple of days to realize that the ulcers were not from the dental bridge but from the chemo treatments. I just put the teeth in a drawer. I can't taste meat and I can eat soup and vegetables without them.

Look on the bright side—beef is expensive big time.

I think that the overall message in this chapter is that chemotherapy brings on oddities to the body that must be dealt with as they appear. After a year and a half of self-observation, I have found that after the completion of the treatment, the side effects are slowly going away or have just sort of ceased to matter. I can't put enough emphasis on the word "slowly." We must be patient.

From Sylvia

Nausea is mostly a thing of the past. It used to be the most feared side effect. I was never sick but had stomach aches from the effects of chemo and other meds. No nausea!

Neuropathy is a problem for many chemo patients. At the first sign of stabbing, burning pain in feet or hands, call the doctor. They will "back off" on the offending chemical in your chemo cocktail and they know which one it is.

Neuropathy is usually permanent and is a nasty reminder (daily) that you survived chemo! I'll take neuropathy. I'm glad I'm alive.

Broccoli Tahini Soup

2 T. olive oil
1 onion, diced small
2 garlic cloves, crushed
1 ½ lb. new potatoes, diced small
1 parsnip, or carrot, peeled, diced small
8 c. vegetable broth
1 lb. broccoli florets, with most of the stem removed
¼ c. fresh dill, chopped
¾ t. cumin
¼ t. cinnamon
¼ t. cayenne pepper
¼ t. cardamom
Salt to taste
½ c. tahini

Heat olive oil at medium heat in soup pot. Add onion, saute 10 minutes, stirring occasionally. Add garlic and carrot or parsnip, stir; add spices; stir and cook about 5 minutes. Add potatoes and broth, bring to a boil, and reduce heat. While the vegetables are simmering, pulse broccoli in food processor until finely chopped. Add broccoli to soup and continue simmering until potatoes and carrot or parsnip is tender. Adjust seasonings to your taste. Whisk in tahini and heat through.

Chicken & Cabbage Soup

4 c. water
3 c. chicken stock
1 can diced tomato
1 stalk celery, sliced
4 green onions, sliced with the green part too
4-5 new potatoes, diced small
1 bay leaf
1 t. salt
½ t. dried thyme
¼ t. fennel or caraway seeds
3 c. finely shredded cabbage
1 c. cubed, cooked chicken
1 T. lemon juice

In a large soup pot, combine first 10 ingredients. Simmer until potatoes are tender. Add cabbage, chicken, and lemon juice and simmer until cabbage is cooked down.

"No misfortune is so bad that whining about it won't make it worse."

> **Jeffrey R. Holland**

"Hope is important because it can make the present moment less difficult to bear. If we believe that tomorrow will be better, we can bear a hardship today."

> **Thich Nhat Hanh**

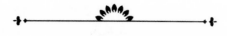

CHAPTER II

Social Aspects

Where I live, in the southeastern United States, ladies have a phrase—"Bless her heart"—which translates to, "I'm glad it's not me." I've heard it applied to me behind my back. "He's doing chemo treatments and lost his hair, bless his heart." I have also heard, "She's skinny as a scarecrow. It must be the cancer treatments, bless her heart."

My wife often says, "These days, cancer seems to touch everyone." I agree with her and I think that one of the reasons for this is that diagnosis procedures are more effective and common than they once were. I think that more and more cancer problems are being found in the early stages where they may be treated effectively.

I have mentioned earlier that something I never understood until I went through the process is that cancer patients who show signs of the side effects of cancer treatments are not always showing signs of the cancer itself. For instance, in my pre-cancer awareness days I can recall seeing people who just looked and felt terrible. In my mind, I just knew it was the cancer that was killing them. I never expected them to live, bless their hearts. I was wrong, though. It was the *treatment* that was making them look and feel that way and once the treatment had done its job, they quickly regained their health and vigor.

The good side of this is that when you are taking the treatment lots of people want to help you and you are treated with kindness. There are many organizations designed to help with any and all of your needs.

I found out a long time before I even got cancer that "when you quit drinking or get sick, you find out who your friends are." Just like right after I quit drinking, a lot of people quit coming around after they heard I had cancer. I don't think this was out of malice but rather because they don't know how to handle my problem on their level. I even noticed that several of my regular customers stopped calling during and after my treatment. I called one client to let her know it was time for some pruning. She replied, "Oh, I have so wanted to call you but I didn't know how it was with your cancer and all." I realized that sometimes people were making their decisions about how to treat me based on ignorance of the facts.

So, one of the things my wife and I did was send out email newsletters to let our friends know how things were progressing. Dekie set up three files because not everyone in every group needed to know the same things: Family, Close friends, John's girlfriends (jokingly—because most of my clients and contacts are women!)

This let people know that I was not dying and things were going as expected or better. The emails also gave the recipients a way to respond unobtrusively. The letter I liked the most was the one that told everyone the PET scan showed that the cancer was gone.

Even six months after my treatments ended, I found out that my two sons hesitated to ask me to help one of them move into his new house "well, you know, because of the cancer thing." I quickly let them know that I was not dead or disabled and after that was straightened out, I was able to show up with a truck and a helper to be of assistance. I think that proved something to them and to me.

Because I am having trouble swallowing due to the radiation on my throat, and because my sense of taste is limited, people seem to feel uncomfortable inviting me (us) for dinner. It's nothing personal. I think that they just hate to ask what I can or cannot eat. When or if they do ask, I may suggest an item or two or I may suggest that they prepare for unimpaired appetites and that I will make do the best I can. It makes me feel self-conscious if others are limiting their dining choices because of my difficulties. My eating rule is "I'll try anything," and I am often surprised when I try something new and it works. It just goes to show,

"Everything is going to be all right."

One thing that we don't want is to overdo things in order to prove a point. Take things slowly for a period during and for a long while after your treatments. This is not to say "don't get any exercise at all," but, for instance, that it may be better to observe a Breast Cancer Run than to participate in it. There will be time for participation later on.

Don't attempt to host elaborate entertainment events during and shortly after your treatments. Admit to yourself that perhaps you need to feel a bit better before such endeavors. Limit your entertainment levels to small efforts that will keep physical and mental stress to a minimum. Before committing yourself to hosting anything, take good inventory of your physical and mental recovery. Recovery is slow and sometimes a lot of us feel like we are Superman and that we can accomplish anything. Sometimes it is better to wait until the healing has progressed to higher levels.

On the other hand, *do* go to concerts or talks or other events that do not involve high demands on your physical abilities. Attend your writer's group or reading club. Go to church or to other sedentary sorts of social events. If you are bald headed, don't worry about it—wear a hat or a wig if it bothers you or tell people that you are supporting solidarity for bald guys. That sort of thing just doesn't matter in the long run. The more jokes you can make about your temporary disabilities and appearances, the better.

My friend Sylvia told me that during her year-long period of chemo treatments, she would force herself to put on her wig and makeup every morning, no matter how she felt. She said that this made her feel a bit more normal and that it was a statement that she was still in charge of her life.

From Sylvia

John, I think you are missing an important element in cancer treatment, especially for women. You are dismissive of hair loss but it is a **big deal** for many, if not most women. After learning they have to undergo chemo I'll bet most women's first question to the doctor is, "Will I lose my hair?"

In not addressing this issue, you aren't giving women the help they need. There are many high quality wigs out there. Others can't tell it's not your own hair. Synthetic wigs are wash and wear while those made from real hair require a beautician's care.

Many women wear scarves or bandanas and look lovely (not me) and a few brave ones go out bald. I wore a bandana once when I felt good enough to go to Tuesday Morning but a woman there asked me if I was going through chemo.

There I was trying to feel normal but the bandana marked me as a cancer patient, so I never went out without my wig again. I admire those who show their baldness as an act of courage but I just wanted to look as much like my old, healthy self as possible. Sorry, I could write a book on this subject.

There is an organization called Look Good Feel Better (lookgoodfeelbetter.org), where local hair dressers and make-up experts give women a makeover, show techniques for tying head scarves and give away cosmetics for free. If you look good you do feel better!

FROM THE JOURNAL

Ulrike Gorgens is the Adult Nurse Practioner. She's slim and she wears boots and I saw her a week ago with her motorcycle helmet. So she got a copy of Requiem today and just as I started to tell her about Kickstand, she started telling me about falling at the entrance to her subdivision because her kickstand foot slipped on a leaf. I therefore decided to stop telling her and let her read it for herself.

(My friend, Dr.) Joel Todino asked several questions. Here are the answers:

The fatigue should begin to dissipate about two weeks after the final chemo treatment which is Wednesday, March 27.

Yes, Joel, 1/6 is code for one more chemo and 6 radiation left.

The taste comes back slowly taking as much as 3 months but different tastes come back before others. Cheese should be early and chocolate will be last. I forgot to specify meat.

I will go to see Dr. Hortman and tell him that I would like to have my teeth finished when it is time to eat cheese crackers. I'm sure he will cooperate.

I will bring the flower pots for your cucumber plants tomorrow.

The doctor is still amazed with the amount of class, style, and stamina that I have exhibited with my treatments. I was in trouble because I lost 5 pounds but I know for sure that is not much. I've talked to at least one person who lost 40 pounds. And I started out 15 pounds overweight on purpose.

I'm going to attribute my success to humor and optimism—both of which improve with practice, and I've been practicing for a long time.

My guys decided that it was too cold and windy to work on the mountain today. It made me happy, too, because I really didn't want to be out in it. I came home and watched a movie. I can concentrate on that these days.

I've learned to go ahead and write these updates because Bob Hicks demands them. One must obey one's father-in-law. Here it is Bob. All is well. I'm going to whup this here cancer.

The tumors are gone.

The doctor said that next week we will make an appointment for six or so weeks in the future to get another PET scan to prove that the system has worked. She feels most confident. We are almost ready to let the healing begin.

john

The above is a sample of a group letter that I sent to my supporters. Looking back at it, I see that all of the information on taste and eating that I was given turned out to be wrong. I never could get any good information on the matter. That's why I kept a food list.

"It takes no more time to see the good side of life than to see the bad."

➤Jimmy Buffett

"You have brains in your head. You have feet in your shoes.
You can steer yourself in any direction you choose.
You're on your own, and you know what you know.
And you are the one who'll decide where to go."

➤Dr. Seuss

CHAPTER 12

End of Treatment

For six weeks I got up at five in the morning and drove about eighty miles to Atlanta for a treatment. One morning I woke up at five, sat up in bed, thought, "wait, yesterday was my last treatment. I don't have to go any- where today." I smiled big, lay back down, and went to sleep. What a wonderful experience that was.

FROM THE JOURNAL

Talk about some journaling. I got depressed and wrote the following which brought me back up again. There's nothing like writing it out and exploring the situation with yourself on paper.

Dealing with it.

It seems like I've been dealing with this thing forever but it's only really been 6 months.

I'm a writer.

I'm paying the bills as fast as I can.

And I haven't been able to get my computer out of the shop for the lack of $75.00. I feel like Fitzgerald having hocked his typewriter but I'm not allowed to get drunk like he was.

There are now 12 more days of treatments facing me. Gas is running about $50.00 per day which covers going to Atlanta and then taking care of job related travel. The job related travel is relegated to the background and shouldn't be because this is what pays for the rest of what all is going on.

And there's not enough time left from the treatments to increase the income or the work load.

Yesterday I felt good all day except that I started the day with insufficient funds to put gas in the truck and even though I ended the day with money in the bank, it just ain't enough.

And a new hospital bill rolls in almost every other day.

Nutrition-wise I'm at the place I didn't want to be. I think the next few weeks will find me getting my nourishment out of a can exclusively. I guess it doesn't really matter, though, because there's no taste at all in anything I eat. None, so I can drink that shit or pour it down a tube and it just doesn't matter.

I guess it doesn't matter, really, that my voice is getting ready to shut down as well. I think the radiational swelling will take its toll in the next week.

Maybe that's where I need to go for a while—just accepting the entire scenario and tucking it all in the back of my brain and pretending that it just doesn't matter. This seems to be the only place to find equanimity. Pretend that it doesn't matter and hope that everyone and everything else leaves me alone.

Here's the thing
If you're not wealthy
And you get sick
And you can't work
You don't get to worry about the sick part because of the work part.

That's why everyone thinks I am doing so well—because I don't have time to worry about or dwell on being sick because I have to spend my energies on getting by. Not getting ahead, not keeping up, but getting by.

And as I write this I can hear my wife in the bed crying. I have no idea what to do about that.

But it is almost over. I can see me feeling really good by the end of April which will be right in time for

business to go wild and things to improve. The weather yesterday was wonderful and really did me a lot of good. I'm glad the weekend is here. I want to feed the plants in the greenhouse and clean the truck. I want to do a lot of things but I'll bet it won't happen.
Almost over...
I keep calling up those words. Almost over...
I didn't mean to jump on Dekie last night but it's Almost Over and that's when stuff like that happens.

I keep going back to Michener's Alaska and the people committing suicide when the winter was Almost Over.

I don't want to go there. I want to be happy that it's almost over and to just relax and let it happen. I don't want to bring down those around me, I want to handle it myself and make it go away. I want to protect those I love who are hurt by what is going on in my life that affects their lives. I just don't know how to do it.

So here is the time for optimism and humor. I said I could write a book about dealing with cancer with optimism and humor so let's let it fly.

I'll bet that there are a lot of people in my situation and that there are a lot of them who don't have as much inner strength as I do in order to handle it. What do I tell them?
Is there a system or a paradigm in which all of the

issues could be packed into a box (so to speak) and just wait until it is over to be dealt with?

That's my new project: A time vault that will move the concerns on to another day when it will be easier to deal with it.

A list, maybe.

A list of all the stuff that can be saved for another day. Put it on the list and relegate it to the future. There, that's pretty funny.

One day in the future, I will feel like dealing with it and it will be easy.

Maybe not easy, but at least not encumbered by the other stresses.
That's it.
A list for June.
yes

A day or two later, I was able to write the following notes:

30
I am realizing what an important part of my life is found in the ritual of snacks. Right now there is no sense in preparing anything. It all tastes like mouldy newspaper. I will be so happy when a good plate of

cheese and crackers tastes like it should. It brings tears to my eyes thinking about it. I hope it's gouda for you. But the optimism holds. I only have one more chemo treatment on Wednesday the 27th. That will be number 7 and done. One more chemo treatment is a piece of cake. J. R. Is going to drive me Monday and Tuesday which will be a nice visit.

All for now. I'm basically happy.
John

And a few days later:

The big news is the final chemo infusion is done over with!!!

When we saw that the little electronic pump that feeds the evil liquid into my veins was empty and that the drip infusion was done, we did a thumbs up and everyone in the bay who had been sharing stories were happy for me. I got tears in my eyes and didn't even try to hide them with masculinity. It was emotional. I'm getting the tears back as I write this. What a trip that was—7 several hour chemical treatments sandwiched in with 35 radiation treatments.

Then I rang the bell and, as Billy would of said, "They stood up and 'plauded'"

Now I only have 4 more radiation treatments. That

will be a piece of cake. I look for some taste to return within the next month and to take 3 months to a year to return fully (according to the people in the chemo bay).

A man and his wife were telling their tales today in the chemo bay and it seems that they had both had bad cancer problems at the same time. He had a bone marrow thing and she had a problem with her spine. He said, "We would come in for treatment together. I'd push her halfway in the wheel chair and then we would switch places." That brings tears to my eyes even now. It was an emotional day. Sweetie drove, of course, as I told you, "Sweetie drives on chemo days."

My friend Randy Eidson will drive me tomorrow morning. I guess Sweetie and I will share the driving on Friday, and Bob Hicks will take care of the Monday detail. Sweetie wants to drive for my final radiation treatment on April 2. I'm looking to sleep late on April 3.
Maybe even until 6 or so.

My weight was down to 176. I'm sure it will go down a few more pounds before the chemo goes away, but my ideal weight is 170 and I had gained up to 185 before starting the treatments, so I think I will be just fine. I don't want to be fat.

All in all, unless something unexpected happens, I

have gotten out of this thing with effects much lighter than I expected. I have not used the feeding tube yet to everyone's amazement and, you know me, I am stubborn enough to be bound and determined to not have to use it at all. If you didn't know me pretty well you wouldn't be getting this here letter.

I guess that's all for now. The tumors have gone the way of the chemo treatments. Outta here. I can't feel them any more and they were most prominent and growing a couple of months ago. My neck is red and burnt from the radiation, but that too shall pass. That reminds me, constipation is also a side effect but I've found a wonderful new item called Phillips Milk of Magnesia. (joke). It really works, just like when I was a kid.
I heard that I could mix it with vodka and have a "Phillips screwdriver." Hehe, just had to leave you with that.

Looking back at the journal entries, I feel so good about having kept up with them. I see things that I had forgotten, such as the really dark spell that came upon me one night.

But, more importantly, I can look back and see the therapeutic effects of the journal writing. It turned out that this one thing—keeping a journal—was very helpful in helping me to organize my thoughts and fears into a format that could be dealt with.

Roasted Asparagus

1 lb. asparagus, tough ends trimmed off
4 t. olive oil
1 T. balsamic vinegar
Salt and pepper to taste

Preheat oven to 425.
Arrange asparagus single layer deep in a roasting pan. Drizzle olive oil over asparagus and toss a bit to coat. Roast for 15-20 minutes, until tender and browned. Toss with vinegar, salt and pepper before serving.

"Well, you can go on looking forward," said Gandalf. "There may be many unexpected feasts ahead of you."

➤**J.R.R. Tolkien**

The Fellowship of the Ring

"The appearance of things changes according to the emotions; and thus we see magic and beauty in them, while the magic and beauty are really in ourselves."

➤**Khalil Gibran**

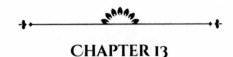

CHAPTER 13

After Effects

FROM THE JOURNAL

The cancer fight: For forty consecutive week days you make it to the clinic in Atlanta for radiation treatments every day and chemo infusions every Wednesday. They are pummelling the body with radioactive poisons and injecting the blood with even more poisons. Now the healing starts—No telling how long it takes. I just hope the sense of taste returns as soon as possible. Now the healing begins.

I asked the doctor, "Is it over? I'm done with the treatments?"

"It's cumulative," he replied. "You have finished the treatments, but the effects of the treatments will progress a bit."

It took a lot of thinking to wrap my brain around those two words, "It's cumulative." I am writing this almost a year after I started my treatments. I am now beginning to understand what "cumulative" means. For a couple of months, things got worse. My throat became stiffer and my taste buds seemed to lose more and more sensitivity. My hair stayed the same for a while and then started growing. I had to learn to shave again. My fingernails started growing and I had to remember to keep them trimmed. I had gotten out of the habit.

A year later I am just beginning to be able to taste and smell things. I realize that I will never again have a normal sense of smell because the trachea operation cut my nose off from air circulation, but for the past several weeks I have noticed that now and then I will walk into the kitchen and smell something cooking. I am finally beginning to taste a variety of things. Just yesterday I found that my taste for Mandarin Orange herbal tea had returned. That made me really happy because this has always been one of my favorite beverages.

Soup with cabbage in it has become a favorite. I was raised in old German traditions and was always a "meat and potatoes" guy. I can remember being rather upset any time there was no meat for the evening meal. One of my most hated words was "vegetarian." Talk about the true meaning of irony—other than a little pork sausage now and then I have no use or taste for red meat, fish, or poultry. I do enjoy poultry stock for soup making and sometimes some well-flavored gravy will make mashed potatoes taste better.

Then there is difficulty swallowing, which I understand is a common problem among throat cancer and laryngectomy victims. So I'm hit with a double whammy. Some things, like stringy meat, barbecue and, strangely enough, some breads, are hard for me to swallow. Certain crackers and chips are the exception.

And I used to love potatoes—mashed, fried, boiled, broiled—you name it. Now, potatoes are merely a conveyance for gravy or ketchup. However, my lovely wife discovered a way to fool me into thinking I was eating mashed potatoes. Check out the recipe for Faux Taters on page 23 to see what I mean! One of the most wonderfully tasty items for me is yellow mustard. Yes, the cheap yellow mustard that goes on hot dogs.

Some other effects I have noticed involve stiffness in my neck and shoulder. I think some is from the radiation and some is from my operation. I tried physical therapy for a while until the insurance funding ran out and it helped a bit, but looking back, I think the recovery just takes time. The stiffness in my neck slowly improves and the turning radius of my head slowly increases.

My speech with the prosthesis steadily improves but I'm not sure how to differentiate improvement due to radiation healing from that due to healing from the operation. I think the speech also improves with time and practice, enabling me to say out loud,

"Everything is going to be all right."

FROM THE JOURNAL

June 29, 2013

So the oncology doctor told me that the results of the PET scan "couldn't have been any better." The cancer is gone. She also said that it would take a loooonnng time to get over the effects of the treatments. I can

live with that—emphasis on "live." Thanks to my sweet wife Dekie Hicks for her loving support and for putting up with me. And thanks to my wonderful family and friends for your help and caring. It means a lot. And Jane Schulz, I love you.

July 18, 2013
Part of my job description is buying lunch for my workers. For the last year or so I have gone inside to order and avoided drive through ordering because at first I didn't have a voice, and then I had a new store bought voice that I didn't trust. Today at Taco Bell inside was crowded and there was no line at the drive through so I decided to take the risk. Guess what!! They understood me and I successfully placed the order.

This may not sound like much to you but it was a red letter day for me.

And these are some of the thoughts that makes it all worthwile:

July 18 2013
Cancer:
When they tell you that you have cancer, it's scary.

And when you find out about the difficult treatments, it's scary.

❖

But after a while, you realize that it's a good thing they found the cancer when they did, because then at least you have a fighting chance.

Those are some of my thoughts on the matter.

And then there are the long range after effects.

My lovely sister, Mary de Wit, is one of my cancer heroes. After going through a number of difficult surgical procedures, she was pronounced cancer free. Mary worked out and dieted and became a physical dynamo. One day in October, she informed me that she was entered in a distance run benefitting breast cancer research.

When I made a remark about how difficult it would be for me to run such a race, she replied with words that I think would apply to any cancer patient:

"You run when you can. When you get to the big hill, you walk."

This statement is brilliant in its suggestion that no matter what, you keep going.

Behold, we know not anything;
I can but trust that good shall fall
At last—far off—at last, to all,
And every winter change to spring.

➤**Alfred Tennyson**

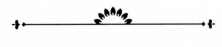

CHAPTER 14

Diet

I was talking with the chemo doctor and his nurse practitioner during my last chemo check up. I asked, "What can you tell me about what I would enjoy eating. My taste is gone. What do your other patients say? Is there a list somewhere? Please give me some information."

The doctor and the nurse looked at each other. I waited for a reply. After a while, they started talking about the weather. That's how I found out that I was on my own, food-wise. I'm not putting them down. I understand now that it's different for everyone, but at the time I was rather frustrated. That's when I decided that I would try everything. My famous statement to my wife (who is a wonderful cook) was, "I'll try anything," and I did. I kept a list of tolerable food in my journal.

From Sylvia:

"Regarding food, I think that will be individual. It was trial-and-error for me because nothing really sounded good and most things didn't taste good, including coffee, my morning lover and wine, my dinner companion. Cold drinks were out; soft foods were in—boiled eggs, yogurt, applesauce, vanilla ice cream, oatmeal and soup. Yes, soup, wonderful soup. I hated Ensure and Boost but tried to drink a little each day. I lost 10 lbs that I didn't have to lose but after treatment gradually found them one at a time. Yes, food is just another of the cancer battles that must be fought."

When I found out that radiation and chemo treatments were going to be a part of my life, my mother talked with a doctor friend of hers who gave me a wonderful piece of advice, "Put on some weight quickly." I am about six feet, two inches tall and I weighed about 170 at that point. I listened to the advice and ate everything in front of me that didn't move. My weight went up about twelve pounds. I guess I topped out at 185 pounds. It was interesting to see what happened to my weight.

At the cancer clinic, whenever I walked into a room for an appointment, the first thing that happened was that I had my blood pressure, temperature, and weight checked. Over the six weeks period I watched my weight go from 185 down to 168. Like one of the doctors had told me, though, the treatment effects are cumulative and my weight kept going down until it reached 162 about five weeks after the final treatment. Then it started going back up. A year after the start of the treatments I weighed in at 177 and everyone who knows me remarks on how healthy I look. I'm going to watch it, though, because I don't want to gain too much more.

Here's another funny dietary thing. I always loved ice cream. I quit drinking alcohol a number of years ago and I think I subconsciously replaced the alcohol with ice cream. One thing I did when I started my daily hour-and-a-half drive to Atlanta was to stop at a well located convenience store right before the interstate ramp. I would get whatever gas I needed, relieve myself, and purchase an ice cream cone. After a couple of weeks of treatments the ice cream no longer had any taste and I switched to Fritos. That lasted for a while and then the Fritos also lost their taste.

I tried Famous Amos chocolate chip cookies. They lasted about a week and then I lost my taste for chocolate. Then things took another twist—my throat started closing down from the radiation. To deal with this I started drinking canned meals for my nutrition. This tasted almost good for a while and then even that bit of taste went away.

I disappeared into my mantra:

"Everything is going to be all right."

I decided that I wouldn't allow the loss of taste to discourage me in my quest to get rid of cancer. I just decided that I would try anything that was put in front of me. My wonderful wife tried so hard to help me find things to eat. I started keeping a list on my iPhone note pad of anything that I found even remotely pleasing. The list ended up looking like this:

CANCER FOOD

Sausage patty and egg
Blue Bell fudge bars
Zucchini

Roasted veggies with vinegar
Eggplant
Pineapple
Pineapple chicken
Cabbage dish
Shrimp and grits
Beets
Balsamic vinegar
Sausage and okra gumbo
Smoked salmon with cream cheese on pumpernickel
Casserole with pasta, Italian sausage and homemade
tomato sauce
Fresh tomato slice with vinaigrette
Cabbage casserole

9/26
lots of taste in Campbell's onion soup
Miso soup
Sylvia's chicken cabbage soup.
Chicken livers
Fried green tomatoes.
Ok I don't taste salt but the canned green beans tasted
salty. (Dekie said she put no salt but did put in a tiny
bit of lemon rind.)
Mary's Smithfield polish kielbasa and andouille sausages
chopped cabbage all cooked together. Excellent

Nov. 3
Ketchup, yellow mustard, Worchestershire sauce and
brown sugar glaze on turkey meat loaf. The yellow
mustard comes through loud and clear.

Roasted butternut squash, sweet potato, chick peas
Cabbage curry
Squash casserole
Roasted butternut squash soup.

12/14/13
broccoli/mushroom casserole.
Harvest moon—Dekie's 52nd birthday. Collards,cheese grits, and roasted asparagus.
Potato and smoked salmon chowder
Creamy broccoli tahini soup.
Avocado shrimp from Micheline

Looking back I see that keeping the list and "trying anything" was my optimism helping me to stay well-fed. I find it most interesting that roasted vegetables became a mainstay for me. It seems that my body was reaching out for what was good for it. I really think the squash casserole was to become my all time favorite.

We joke about the food thing by saying that before chemo, God made two lists—one of everything I loved and another of everything I hated.

After chemo, He switched the lists.

It's been a year and a half at this writing and I've learned what I like and what I don't. I keep trying new things, too. I can offer guidance to others in this area, but the best thing I can say is, try anything and remember what you could eat and what you couldn't. And remember:

"Everything is going to be all right."

If I can stop one heart from breaking,
I shall not live in vain;
If I can ease one life the aching,
Or cool one pain,
Or help one fainting robin
Unto his nest again,
I shall not live in vain.

➤**Emily Dickinson**

CHAPTER 15

On Caregiving
by Dekie Hicks

When John received his cancer diagnosis, I was dismayed, and scared. I knew that I would be his major caregiver, and I have to admit, one of the first things I wondered was, "How gross is this going to get?"

As it turned out, nothing was too gross! It was, however, tiring and weird. The hardest part of the entire journey for me was dealing with everything between his surgery, which was major and tricky, and the time when he was healed enough to have the voice prosthesis installed, a period of approximately five months. John needed to use a nasal feeding tube for part of this time because he couldn't swallow any hard food as his throat healed. I had to pump his medical grade, Ensure-like food down this tube, which required an amazing amount of physical strength. We quickly came up with some jokes about the process, such as realizing a bit late that we could cut the stuff with water, making it easier to pump. Duh! Or laughing at peoples' reactions at the grocery store. He was quite the sight, striding down the aisles with that tube swinging in the air.

During this time, John couldn't speak, so he communicated either by writing everything down or by text messaging and emailing. For a long time after the prosthesis was installed, we found scraps of paper all over the house and in the car, with entire one-sided conversations to read again. We also had some arguments via texting that are funnier in retrospect than they were at the time.

It wasn't long after the surgery when people began to comment to me that I was doing a great job of taking care of him, and dealing with the difficulties presented during this time. I remember being a bit astounded that they would notice these things, much less remark on them. Because it seemed to me that I was merely doing what had to be done, and I had a hard time envisioning myself acting in any other way than what I was already doing. I mean, I could imagine other courses of action—refusing to take over the bulk of communicating with the outside world, or pawning off pumping the formula down his feeding tube onto someone else. But it never occurred to me to actually engage in any of these alternate courses of action.

When people would compliment me on my caregiving, I often responded with, "Oh, but John makes it easy! He isn't a jerk!" And I would say to him, "Thank you for not being an ass. If you were, all of this crap would be SO much more difficult to deal with!" Even during his lowest point emotionally, which was Christmas of 2012, the very end of his recuperation from surgery, when he was so tired of not being able to talk, he was still respectful toward me, and others.

All of this ordeal reminded me of a story my father had told me, years before I even knew John, about a colleague of his who was suffering from bone cancer. This gentleman called my father up and invited him to lunch, warning my dad not to be too shocked by his appearance. My father was shocked, but continued on with the lunch, and this is the story that came out of that lunch:

After the usual pleasantries we began catching up on all that had happened in the intervening two or more decades during which we had not been in contact. We recalled 1953 when we were both in the same law firm and I had come all the way from New York to attend his wedding.

He told me of his travails in the finance business, his rise to riches and fall through bankruptcy, his recovery and return to substantial wealth. But most of all we talked about his health. He had developed bone cancer and for years had been going to various clinics throughout the country—MD Anderson, Sloan-Kettering, Mayo and some place in Arkansas—all without remission. He told of his three children, one of whom had had severe developmental difficulties. He commented that he was unable to decide whether he was happy to have his wits about him so he could reflect on his miserable condition or whether he should die and pave the way for the happiness of others.

I mustered the courage to ask how his wife was. I did not know whether she was doing well, divorced, still alive, or what. I was comforted in the belief that I accurately recalled her first name although I have totally forgotten her maiden name.

He replied: "Well, Bob, I am glad you asked about her. I find a great relief in telling you she seems fine in spite of my condition. About a year ago we were sitting in the glassed-in porch of our house during a very slight snowfall in February. I was drinking a cup of coffee and said in a very complaining, belligerent voice that I could not understand why I could not get a decent cup of hot coffee in my own home. I am sure the tone of my voice was most hostile.

She turned to me and told me to look her directly in the eye . . .

She said: "Ed, I loved you when we got married, I loved you when we had our three children, I loved you through those years when we had so much trouble with our difficult one, I loved you when you made all that money in New York and still loved you when you lost everything, including our home, through bankruptcy. I love it that you recovered financially and we seem to be on easy street in that way, and I am deeply sorry you have cancer, deeply sorry you seem not to have been able to find remission, although you have done everything possible to do so. I love you enough to say from my heart that I wish I could trade places with you, suffer your health burdens and give you my vigor. I plan on living with you until one of us dies, but . . .

*"Ed, you **are** going to be nice to me. I do not ever want to hear that tone of voice again—do you understand?"*

"Bob, you cannot realize what a sense of relief came over me. When she commanded me to look her directly in the eye, I felt terror strike my heart. Was she going to tell me I had finally gone too far? I thanked God she gave me the opportunity to redeem myself. And I believe I have . . .

"She is still with me.'

The reason I have remembered this story for so long is I am most impressed with the lady's refusal to be treated badly, with how she stood up for herself when her husband was being a jerk, and did not let his terrible illness stop her from saying what had to be said.

I consider myself lucky that I never had to have that conversation with John.

And so, I would say to all caregivers that you deserve to be treated kindly no matter how crappy the patient is feeling, no matter how scared everyone is. It is okay for everyone to have the occasional bad moment, or a short spate of complaining and venting, but do not allow it to continue. Absolutely, you have the right to insist on fair treatment.

Which brings me to my final point. Take care of yourself. For me, this meant visiting friends and going out to dinner to kick up my heels a bit while John was in the hospital recuperating from the neck surgery. The surgery to remove the tumors had taken seven hours. I waited, along with various friends and family, all of that time in the waiting area, but once the surgeon gave us the good news that the surgery had been successful, and once John was awake and settled in his room, I headed out to a nice dinner at a local restaurant! After all, I had something to celebrate, and it turned out that an old family friend was having a birthday party, so I joined right in. I knew John was surrounded by skilled nurses who could care for him much better than I could at that moment.

Later on in the journey, when he was hooked up to the chemo infusion drip, I left him there and visited friends I hadn't seen in a while, or went for walks with my camera, or just drove around. Throughout everything, I continued teaching tai chi and working out to maintain my physical strength, which I needed more than I anticipated. I cooked treats for myself, and if John couldn't eat them, oh well! I even took a trip with my father during John's chemo. This trip had already been scheduled, and rescheduled again, and finally, I just said, "Oh, screw it! Papa and I are going on this trip now, before you get really knocked back by the chemo." And my father and I had a good time! I knew John had other people he could call on while I was gone.

Now it is coming up on two years since the final radiation treatment. We made it through and both of us have learned much about illness and its attendant issues. The next time I am called into caregiving mode—because I will be; it's the nature of life—I will know how to take care of myself and make the best of what is happening. Most of all, I now truly know that:

"Everything is going to be all right!"

Jane's Peach Crunch

3-4 c. sliced peaches, or other fruit
1 c. Bisquick
1 c. sugar
1 egg
3/4 stick butter, melted

Mix Bisquick, sugar and egg until crumbly. Put fruit in pie plate and spread or drop the batter over the fruit. Drizzle the butter over all.

Bake at 350 for 20-25 minutes, until bubbly and browned.

About John P. Schulz

I lost my vocal cords a while back due to throat cancer. The laryngectomy sent me on a quest to find and learn to use my new, altered voice. Now I am able to talk thanks to a small and neat new prosthesis and I think it's funny that through all of the changes, I have found that my writing has become my new voice.

A few years ago when I was first told that I had cancer, I was immediately concerned with many questions and fears. The cancer center gave me a book that didn't really help, so I decided that I would keep a journal throughout my treatment time and later write the book that I would have liked to have had at that time. That's where *Sweetie Drives on Chemo Days* came from. I have written it to help people understand a bit of what goes on during cancer treatment, and to calm a few fears. I am a firm believer in the curative powers of optimism. I do believe that, "Everything is going to be all right."

I am also the author of *Requiem for a Redneck* and *Redemption for a Redneck*—funny and sensitive novels portraying the lives and doings of folks from the north Georgia hills. I am working on the third part of the trilogy, *Resurrection for a Redneck*. I can be found online at johnschulzauthor.com, johntheplantman.com, and John P. Schulz Author on Facebook.

I have an English Education degree from the University of Georgia and am very happily married to the lovely Dekie Hicks.

CPSIA information can be obtained at www.ICGtesting.com
Printed in the USA
LVOW11s0026230315

431599LV00003B/4/P